PRAISE FOR DR. CLEMENT

"Dr. Clement possesses the experience and knowledge to spearhead the emerging field of authentic health care."

—Coretta Scott King

"Dr. Clement and the Hippocrates Institute, conducting clinical research on hundreds of thousands over the last half century, clearly uncovered the fraud that is most often called 'Natural Supplements.' Read this, take it to heart, and tell all of your friends about it."

—Victoras Kulvinskas, MS,
Cofounder Hippocrates Health Institute

SUPPLEMENTS EXPOSED

The Truth They Don't Want You
to Know About Vitamins,
Minerals, and Their Effects
on Your Health

BRIAN R. CLEMENT, PhD

*Director of the Hippocrates
Health Institute*

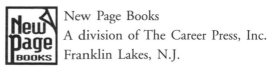

New Page Books
A division of The Career Press, Inc.
Franklin Lakes, N.J.

SUPPLEMENTS EXPOSED
Edited andTypeset by Kara A. Kumpel
Cover design by Lucia Rossman/DigiDog Design
Printed in the U.S.A. by Courier

To order this title, please call toll-free 1-800-CAREER-1 (NJ and Canada: 201-848-0310) to order using VISA or MasterCard, or for further information on books from Career Press.

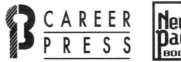

The Career Press, Inc., 3 Tice Road, PO Box 687,
Franklin Lakes, NJ 07417
www.careerpress.com
www.newpagebooks.com

Cataloging-in-Publication Data Available Upon Request

ACKNOWLEDGMENTS

Throughout the years I have had the privilege of working in the field of complimentary healthcare. My one consistent nemesis has been the fraud that is called the supplement industry. Several years ago, my colleague, Dr. Scott Treadway, sent me his written thoughts on a potential book we should write exposing this fallacy. He threw me the ball and I fortunately began to work with researcher and editor Randall Fitzgerald, who was an essential part of the development of this powerful manuscript.

During the time it took to investigate and develop a concise and clear portrayal of the history and derailment of nutrients in a pill we unveiled extraordinary disparities between whole-food, naturally occurring supplements and those made in chemical laboratories. Both Treadway, who is a well-known manufacturer of proper supplements, and Fitzgerald, a renowned investigative journalist, brought me volumes of data and science tracing the deceptive methods used by pharmaceutical and mega supplement companies, showing how they deceive the general public.

The efforts put forth by my two colleagues made this a landmark book in the field of human health. It is my hope that millions share our shock at how the majority of so-called natural supplements have often mistreated us. It is my objective to shine a bright light on the importance of good nutrient intake and squelch the stereotypical belief that all nutrients are created equal. In our daily research here at the Hippocrates Health Institute, we further this knowledge and solidify its reality.

Thank you to all that helped me make *Supplements Exposed* the first book that honestly reveals one of the most precarious misunderstandings of today. Without the efforts of those I have mentioned and others, such as my wife, Dr. Anna Maria Gahns-Clement, and my four children, Daly, Danielle, Gail, and Blake, who often participated in the hours it took to assemble this publication, it would not have come to pass.

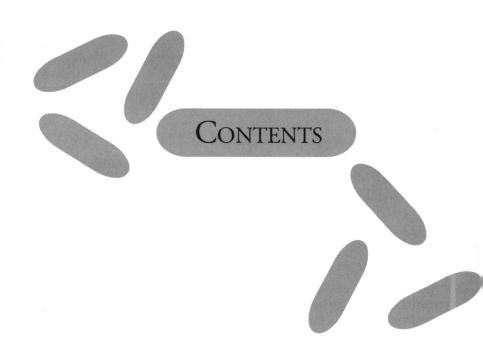

CONTENTS

FOREWORD

BY VALERIE V. HUNT

This monumental book is more than just a brilliant survey and critique on supplements such as vitamins, minerals, and fatty acids. Next to psychology, more words have been written about food needs than on any other subject. These are often written from personal experience, from shoddy multivariable research, and some from rigid research methods meeting the scientific criteria (controllable, repeatable, and limited in concept).

Dr. Clement, with his rich academic and research background in authentic science, combined with extensive research at the Hippocrates Institute, gives this book abstracted, "digested," integrated, far-reaching information, written in clear literary form. These should be the last words on our choices of habits to nourish ourselves as we communicate with our world of living, evolving plant life and mineral elements. Those of you who are acquainted with my research know that I have cracked the "cosmic egg," the next frontier in medicine and health, with scientific evaluation, diagnosis, and treatment of the *bioenergy field*, or human frequency, as described in my book *Infinite Mind: Science of the Human Vibrations of Consciousness*. The bioenergy field at last demonstrates that the primary life goals of the future will be *health* and not *absence of disease*.

It is therefore appropriate that I be affiliated with the best nutritional concepts as those presented by Dr. Clement, whose aim is the initiation and maintenance of a healthy life through food rather than recovery from disease and malfunction.

What Is Life?

Our earliest beliefs were that life came from the proper chemical soup where cells multiplied, grew, and organized to create a living, dynamic organism. This belief was incorrect—nothing happened until there was an electrical charge to start the chemical changes. Life is first and basically the result of electromagnetic charges. These electrical charges come from atoms, the smallest-mass substance in the body. Physics tells us that when the atom splits, it releases energy, which is the life force provoking continued growth and repair. In warm-blooded organisms such as humans, this is metabolism, which maintains life. The atomic energy released is in positive and negative charges, or ions. The positive ions recirculate in the body as free radicals looking for negative ions to reestablish the atom. As we all know, these radicals damage cells until reintegrated with negative ions. At the same time, the negative ions migrate to the surface of the body and become the auric field. These negative ions do not quickly escape, because the surface of the body, the skin, is positively ionized to hold them radiating around the anatomy.

My young nephew calls this energy "that fuzzy stuff hanging around the body which you see when you squint."

I found that the reason we have not recorded these vibrations before is because they are so tiny, in microvolt (one millionth of a volt). The available instruments were developed to test energy in millivolts only (thousandths of a volt), such as the energy of the brain, the muscles, and the heart.

I developed equipment to measure this energy in microvolts, which is like a shadow, but microscopically very real.

This leads me to describe how all mass is composed of atoms—metal, rock, wood, manmade substances, and so on, but the organized manifestation of these atoms is static. They are not living and changing—

they are just radiating a narrow, limited field. We sense these vibrations but our field only reacts blandly. With living plants, animals, trees, and air—all dynamic vibrating substances—we dynamically transact, meaning our bioenergy field selects the field vibrations it likes best. Furthermore, our auric fields are organized for each individual by her/his emotions to perpetuate her/his life and health, utilizing and giving her/him pleasure.

Now with an organized selective field we accept and reject some vibrations based upon our experience. So habit patterns from core experiences goof up the ideal that nature gave us—good health does not occur when making bad choices.

Such information about our transactions with the vibrations of the earth leads us directly to Dr. Clement's insights that living, growing things, and plant life, have the live vibrations that keep us healthy, vital, and transacting within this world of information and balance.

Dr. Clement states that the body's vibrational system has the correct choices built into its field of communication. It knows the difference between the pure and natural substances and the synthetic ones that do not vibrate like the living body.

The author has shown us that much of the research on nutritional needs is connected to disease. Film of Kirlian photography, or light-beam chromatography, shows us radiating vibrations from living food. Such techniques do not show the dramatic transaction between the human aura and living foods. The "zip code" Dr. Clement speaks about is the transaction between similar vibrations in the food and body, which fosters absorption of natural chemicals.

Bioavailability of natural vitamins with their naturally occurring associated factors and trace substances are patterns of compatible nutro-biovibrations.

I loved his criticism of double-blind studies that do not take into account the accurate reactions of people. Hippocrates' extensive study of individual nutritional history gives much greater accuracy. Dr. Clement wisely recommends an expanded nutritional program to ensure adequacy and the listing of food sources by new criteria, the Naturally Occurring Standard, or NOS.

Soon I hope my Bioenergy Fields Monitor will be commercially available to check the nutritional transactions of each person beyond the general information of age, gender, dietary health, and stress levels.

I have written forewords for numerous frontier books, but nothing has given me more pleasure than to have been asked to write one for *Supplements Exposed: The Truth They Don't Want You to Know About Vitamins, Minerals, and Their Effects on Your Health.*

I believe this book will be translated in many languages. I thank you, Brian, for your contribution to the world with this small encyclopedia of information, and for your enlightening me on this subject.

With appreciation,
Valerie V. Hunt, EdD in Science Education, RPT
Professor Emeritus, UCLA, Department of Physiological Science
Director of Research, BioEnergy Fields Foundation 501(c)3

INTRODUCTION

NATURE'S PROMISE BETRAYED

If you have ever consumed vitamins at any time in your life—and two-thirds of us have, according to health surveys—you have probably unwittingly bought into one of the most enduring and toxic myths to ever shape public health consciousness.

You have been led to believe that the vitamin supplements you take to fortify your body against illness and disease are both safe and effective. You have been told that these supplements are nature's own natural ingredients packaged in condensed form as a prescription for wellness. You may have even felt that the $22 billion—that's right, $22 *billion*—we spend each year in the United States alone on nutritional supplements is money well invested to protect the public health.

In this book, you will learn how these and many other cherished ideas we hold about nutrition are a dangerous collection of myths and half-truths based on adherence to a synthetic belief system that has led our culture far astray of nature's promise and potential for bestowing health and healing.

The primary problem identified within these pages is that most vitamins sold throughout the world are synthetics, created in laboratories owned or controlled by pharmaceutical companies, and these companies apply the same manufacturing standards and processes to vitamins that they do to prescription and over-the-counter drugs. At least 95 percent of all vitamins manufactured today contain some synthetic ingredients, according to the Organic Consumer's Association.

Manufacturers maintain that their synthetic chemical vitamins concocted in laboratories are identical and just as effective as the naturally occurring vitamins produced in plants by nature. This book will challenge that contention in numerous ways, based on natural principles, science, observed human health impacts, and consumer safety.

Synergy means two or more chemicals or compounds interacting to produce effects more powerful than any one can create by itself. Synergy is a fundamental principle of nature, and a fact that the prevailing synthetics belief system, with its emphasis on isolating "magic bullet" molecules, chooses to ignore at our peril.

In fact, no human can live solely on isolated, synthetic nutrients; we must eat foods created by nature in order to survive. What is it in nature that creates life-sustaining foods and food nutrition that cannot be constructed or replicated by man? Although few of us ponder this great mystery in our practical day-to-day existence, it is an essential factor for both health and life, which are inextricably related.

Although scientists can create seawater with exactly the same chemical structure as natural seawater, when you put a saltwater fish in this synthetic environment, the fish does not thrive or stay as healthy as it does in its natural surroundings. *Reefkeeping*, an online magazine for marine aquarists, points out how synthetic seawater is "an imperfect substitute for what is the perfect medium for marine animal growth, pure oceanic seawater." Some chemists will still try to convince you that seawater is just sodium chloride added to H_2O and that synthetic seawater has an identical chemical structure to natural seawater. But in practice, as aquarium experts note, seawater "is a complex and incompletely understood mixture of virtually every substance that has graced the face of the Earth." These substances create a synergy that nurtures and sustains marine life.

What is it in natural seawater that sustains marine life and creates a force that synthetics produced by humans cannot duplicate? It is the same principle of life-force, the same type of synergy from complex nutrient cofactors, that we find naturally occurring in the foods of nature that nurture and sustain our own forms of life. That life force is one of the themes of this book.

Scientists have never successfully created an apple from scratch in a laboratory. Only nature has proven its ability to produce apples. As the scientist Carl Sagan once aptly put it, "if you want to make an apple pie from scratch, you must first create the universe."

By the same token, neither can science create synthetic nutrients that exactly duplicate or replace naturally occurring nutrients. This book is concerned with the consequences, the impact on your health, when scientific arrogance in the form of a synthetics belief system attempts to impose its will, fueled by inaccurate assumptions, as a substitute for the experience and wisdom of nature.

Mainstream marketing of vitamins and minerals continues to promote the myth among consumers that nutrients can be isolated individually from one another and synthesized in a laboratory to give us the same health benefits as nutrients found working together in organic fruits and vegetables. This is the "magic bullet" mindset that remains the centerpiece of our culture's synthetics belief system. It is a fatally flawed point of view, as this book will demonstrate.

Consumer safety also figures prominently in the superiority of natural versus synthetic supplements. Besides the potentially toxic synthetic colorings (extracted from coal tar), synthetic flavorings, and other additives placed into "nutritional" supplements, many manufacturers of soft-gel vitamins add partially hydrogenated soybean oil. Yes, you read that accurately! The same oils that have been linked as a cause of cardiovascular disease, strokes, and heart attacks are sometimes added as filler to vitamins sold in health food stores.

Did you know that 90 percent of the vitamin C manufactured in the world today is synthetic, and nearly all of that comes from China? Within the past decade, four pharmaceutical companies in mainland China emerged to control the global vitamin C market, though what they are producing is really just ascorbic acid. (The difference between real vitamin C and ascorbic acid will be made clear in a later chapter.) As for the impact on consumer safety of having one nation dominate an important part of the vitamin market, especially in the wake of the melamine contamination of food emanating from China, only time will tell.

Even when conscientious consumers try to avoid synthetics by looking for the word *natural* on a vitamin label, there is no guarantee that *natural* is what they get. The word *natural* has been abused and diluted for so long that it has lost much of its intended meaning, thanks largely to marketing manipulation and political shenanigans on the part of synthetics manufacturers.

Under current law, a vitamin marketed as natural only has to contain 10 percent of genuinely natural, plant-derived ingredients—the other 90 percent of ingredients can be synthetic. If a product contains even one carbon atom, it can legally be called 100-percent organic. These deceptions, too, are a subject of this book.

When we say *natural* or *whole-food* supplements on these pages, we are referring to vitamins and other products that contain the complete complex of micro-nutrients (both identified and unidentified) exactly as they exist in nature. For example, take the nutrient beta-carotene. Synthetic compounds marketed as beta-carotene are usually made from acetylene gas and are isolated molecules.

In nature, beta-carotene is never found isolated and alone, but is part of a large family of carotenoids. So when we find beta-carotene in carrots and tomatoes, we also find alpha-carotene and gamma-carotene and a host of others that all play roles in a synergistic process. By isolating beta-carotene from its extended family of supporting antioxidants and micro-nutrients, synthetic vitamin manufacturers have stripped away many of the health benefits.

It is no wonder that when medical studies have tested the effectiveness of some well-known curative nutrients in preventing illness and disease, their results have sometimes been negative because their producers used synthetic rather than naturally occurring nutrients. The most recent example of researchers reaching a dead end in experiments using synthetics came in research that attempted to identify the role of nutrients in cancer prevention. A June 2009 article in the journal *Clinical Nutrition Insight* reviewed a series of studies that used synthetic supplements and concluded that "nutrition researchers have probably oversimplified the complex relationships between diet and cancer." They have placed too much emphasis on trying to isolate specific bio-active nutrients and not enough attention "to complex mixtures of bio-active compounds." In other words, when it comes to disease prevention, synthetics are no substitute for pure foods. This flawed methodology and fixation on isolating nutrients and making synthetic versions of them is like trying to see a flower but only observing a petal.

As for the bio-availability (your body's absorption) of natural versus synthetic vitamins, there is once again no contest. Your body knows the difference, even though synthetics are designed to try and trick it. Natural nutrients are absorbed readily because we are biologically programmed to recognize the naturally occurring compounds as genuine nutrients. Isolated chemical or synthetic "nutrients," on the other hand, are immediately put on hold by the body until it can determine the cofactors needed to enable their availability. This highly complex process begins with the analysis of the chemical substance and includes determining what resources from its own stores it has and is able to provide in an effort to convert the chemical supplement into a usable form. As you will learn in a later chapter, 50 percent of every synthetic supplement is automatically rendered useless by the body, leaving only 50 percent for possible conversion. Furthermore, there is no guarantee that any, or this entire half, will be converted; it is based solely on an individual's specific resources. Synthetic supplements on the whole are no more than *potential* sources of "nutrition."

A good case in point is synthetic vitamin E, which has been shown in numerous studies to possess half or as little as one-third of the biologically active impact that natural vitamin E has on the human body. Cambridge University Professor Isobel Jennings, a pioneer nutritional researcher, made this point in her book *Vitamins in Endocrine Metabolism*: "Synthetic vitamins, prepared from chemicals instead of nature, are frequently less active biologically than their natural counterparts, thereby reducing any beneficial effect they may have."

Synthetic vitamins are like the images we see in mirrors. They may look exactly like the real thing, just as chemists claim they do when comparing the molecular structure of synthetic and natural molecules under microscopes. But much like the mirror images we see, which cannot function actively except to mimic our movements, synthetic vitamins do not function the same way as the natural chemical compounds they were designed to mimic.

A better reflection of the difference between natural and synthetic comes when we view how these respective molecules react to a polarized beam of light. When passing through a natural vitamin, light always bends to the right because of its molecular rotation. This is why the letter "d," standing for "dextro" and meaning "right," will sometimes appear on labels. By contrast, light rays passing through synthetic vitamins split: One bends to the right, the other to the left, which is why "dl," standing for "dextro" and "levo," which means *left*, sometimes can be found as an identifier on labels.

Synthetic vitamin manufacturers want you to believe there is no difference between synthetic and natural products because the synthetics are cheaper to produce and thus carry a much higher profit margin. It is that simple. It is the triumph of profits over health, and most people in the industrialized countries of the world have unknowingly bought into that value system.

It would be wonderful and certainly ideal if we got all of the essential nutrients beneficial to our health directly from our fruits and vegetables. But the soils most crops are grown in have lost many nutrients in the past few decades as a result of poor farming practices, while even more nutrients are stripped from foods through refining and processing.

Even with organic food crops, which are always preferable to non-organics because they contain higher levels of phytochemical nutrients and low if any levels of pesticides, there is a loss of nutrients during the time between harvest and consumption. There is an even greater nutrient loss if the foods are cooked as opposed to eating them raw. As a result, the U.S. Department of Agriculture (USDA), based on a survey of 21,500 people, found that not a single person consumes 100 percent of the USDA's Recommended Daily Allowance of nutrients from the foods they eat.

So we do need some vitamin and mineral supplementation to satisfy our bodily needs and to maintain an optimum level of health. The real question is whether we consumers will make informed choices about supplements even after learning how superior naturally occurring nutrients are to synthetics.

That is why a case is made for the creation of a Naturally Occurring Standard (NOS), a supplements label that will clearly state if a vitamin or other product comes directly from—and is composed entirely of—compounds derived from the plants themselves. An NOS symbol will help eliminate the confusion about what is genuinely natural as opposed to partly or wholly synthetic.

We are a culture awash with myths, misinformation, and misconceptions about the roles that nutrition and supplementation play or should play in our lives.

You may be one of those people who still believes that if you just eat a balanced diet, whatever that is and however it is defined, you will never really need to consume supplements to maintain your health. Or you may have accepted without question the advertising claims that all vitamins are created equal in their benefits and vary in effect only with dosage levels. Even if you have doubts about some of the advertising claims, you may continue taking supplements in the hope that the old adage "better safe than sorry" will come true. Or perhaps you hope that whatever nature can do, even in the realm of nutrition, science can do better—if not today then someday soon.

This book is addressed to all of you.

Nature gave us a promise. It was the promise of good health and a long life if we use its nutrients wisely as our medicine. The betrayal of this promise by the synthetics belief system has been one of civilization's crowning healthcare disappointments. May the revelations on these pages contribute to bringing our relationship to nature back into its rightful and proper balance so that access to health-giving nutrients and supplementation once again becomes our birthright.

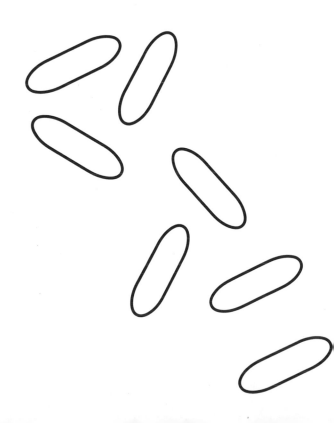

PART I

THE FOUR VITAMIN MISCONCEPTIONS

CHAPTER 1

MISCONCEPTION #1: FOOD CONTAINS ALL THE VITAMINS YOU NEED

Some physicians disparage vitamin use by telling patients that "vitamins only produce expensive urine." Other so-called experts have tried to reassure us that we simply need to eat a balanced diet to get all the nutrients our bodies need.

We even have the 2005 Dietary Guidelines for Americans prepared by two U.S. Government agencies—the Department of Agriculture and the Department of Health and Human Services—telling us to follow this advice about vitamins and food:

> Nutrient needs should be met primarily through consuming foods. Foods provide an array of nutrients (as well as phytochemicals, antioxidants, etc.) and other compounds that may have beneficial effects on health. Supplements may be useful when they fill a specific identified nutrient gap that cannot or is not otherwise being met by the individual's intake of food. Nutrient supplements cannot replace a healthful diet.

In an ideal world, all of this advice would be common sense and would be worth following. But, as you probably know, we do not live in an ideal world—not by any stretch of the imagination—and that is certainly the grim reality when it comes to the availability and quality of the nutrients that we depend upon for optimal health.

We must start with a simple biological fact of life: Vitamins and minerals are essential to human health, and the human body is unable to manufacture most of what it needs. These nutrients must be obtained from the foods that we eat and the supplements we take derived from food.

Once upon a time the soils that grew our food crops naturally contained the nutrients needed by the human body. Today, most organic farm soils contain only 2- to 4-percent organic matter when they should have more than 20-percent organic matter. Most foods used to be eaten fresh soon after harvesting, so these nutrients were largely preserved for absorption. That began to change during the 20th century with the introduction of pesticides, herbicides, and other synthetic chemical contaminants, along with the widespread processing of foods containing added preservatives and other additives.

The mineral depletion of our soils and food crops has been a source of grave concern since at least 1936, when a warning about the problem appeared in a U.S. Senate committee report known as Document 264. Although this was not an official government report or study, but a reprint of a mainstream media article submitted into the record by Senator Duncan Fletcher (D-FL), it nonetheless represented an emerging perspective about the depletion of our soils. Here is an excerpt:

> Most of us today are suffering from certain dangerous diet deficiencies which cannot be remedied until the depleted soils from which our foods come are brought into proper mineral balance. Foods, fruits, vegetables and grains that are now being raised on millions of acres of land that no longer contain enough of certain needed minerals, are starving us no matter how much of them we eat.
>
> Leading authorities state that 99 percent of the world's people are deficient in these minerals, and that a marked deficiency in any one of the more important minerals actually results in disease. Any upset of the balance or any considerable lack of one or another element, however microscopic the body requirement might be, and we

sicken, suffer, and shorten our lives. Lacking vitamins, the system can make some use of minerals; but lacking minerals, vitamins are useless.

Fast-forward this soil depletion process a half-century to 1992 and the first United Nations Conference on Environment and Development, known as the Earth Summit, held in Brazil. That meeting of 108 heads of state was presented with a document prepared by agricultural experts showing the extent to which nutrients had been removed from crop soils worldwide. The estimates were far worse than anyone had previously suspected.

During the 20th century, according to this report, about 85 percent of all nutrients had been depleted from the crop soils of North America. Asia and South America lost 76 percent of soil nutrients. Africa lost 74 percent, and Europe experienced a 72-percent decline. These nutrients were stripped from the soil by fertilizers, pesticides, herbicides, farming practices, irrigation, and other human-induced causes.

At least 90 of these depleted nutrients are considered essential to human health, including 60 minerals and 16 vitamins that are crucial to proper immune-system functioning. Now consider what happens when foods grown in these anemic soils are then processed by the large food-processing corporations and larded with synthetic chemical preservatives, colorings, and other additives. Nutrient levels are reduced once again by 80 percent, and more, in the case of both minerals and vitamins. By the time these foods are then subjected to high heat during cooking, which reduces nutrient levels still further, not much nutrient value is left for the human body to absorb.

Just between the years 1973 and 1997, the U.S. Department of Agriculture reported that nutrients measured in every single category of vegetables grown in the United States fell dramatically. Calcium levels in broccoli dropped 53 percent during that period, thiamine fell 35 percent, and niacin plummeted 29 percent. All of the vegetable measurements for onions, carrots, and a long list of others showed similar sharp declines in essential nutrients.

As if this extensive loss of nutrients at every step of the food-growing and processing chain did not provide ammunition enough for the need to supplement our diets, we now know that few people are meeting even the minimum dietary guidelines for the consumption of beneficial fruits and vegetables. The U.S. Centers for Disease Control and Prevention reported on March 15, 2007, that less than one-third of U.S. residents consume the government's recommended daily intake of fruits and vegetables. Only 27 percent of adults, based on a sampling of 305,000 adults, eat vegetables in large enough quantities each day to absorb any of the vitamins and minerals that help to guard the body against chronic illnesses and diseases.

It is no wonder that science studies are now beginning to generate evidence for a direct link between these vitamin and mineral deficiencies and a range of maladies. A 2005 study titled "A Double-Blind, Placebo-Controlled Exploratory Trial of Chromium Picolinate in Atypical Depression" in the *Journal of Psychiatric Practice*, for example, examined 113 people ranging in age from 18 to 65 years old and found that those exhibiting symptoms of depression also tested positive for a deficiency in chromium, a trace mineral normally found in food crops. When chromium supplements were given to those test subjects with depression, their symptoms showed "significantly greater improvements," according to the study authors, John Docherty and others. For the estimated 30 million people, in America alone, who have suffered from depression, these results should be a beacon of hope.

Other science studies have highlighted a range of health benefits from vitamin and mineral supplementation. Low levels of vitamin B5 have been linked to symptoms of arthritis, and vitamin B3 (niacin) has been shown to improve joint flexibility and to reduce joint inflammation. Many people with arthritis also have severe calcium deficiencies. The Rheumatoid Disease Foundation touts boron supplements to help relieve rheumatoid arthritis and osteoarthritis, which afflict 20 million people in the United States alone.

Research has shown vitamins E and C and beta-carotene to be key to eye health, and numerous epidemiological studies have linked vitamin E and beta-carotene to reduced incidence of heart disease. *The Journal of Nutrition* has reported studies showing that multivitamins can reduce myocardial infarction. Nine randomized controlled trials found that chromium supplements enhance insulin sensitivity and improve blood sugar control in diabetics. And the list of other potential health benefits goes on and on.

Some vitamins and minerals, such as selenium and vitamins C and E, play the role of antioxidants in the human body and act synergistically to become our front-line defense against cancer and heart disease. "The fact that not even the recommended daily dosage can be attained by a regular diet leads to the need for antioxidant supplementation," observed Yousry Naguib, a product manager of Soft Gel Technologies of Los Angeles, in comments he made to a trade industry journal in 2004. "Antioxidants tend to work as a team in synergistic fashion. They constitute an interlinked defense system that protects against disease associated with oxidative stress."

Many medical experts are beginning to speak out in the strongest possible terms about the benefits of supplementation. "We now have a substantial body of data showing that if everyone took a few supplements every day, they could significantly lower their risk of a multitude of serious diseases," reports Dr. David Heber, a founding director of the Center for Human Nutrition at the University of California, Los Angeles (UCLA). During his testimony before a committee of the U.S. Congress in 2002, in which he detailed his research into the use of botanical supplements to treat cancer and other diseases, Dr. Heber made these observations about the role of vitamins in our lives:

> Modern humans evolved about 50,000 years ago in Africa in a veritable Garden of Eden where our genes were in equilibrium with a varied and colorful diet of plant foods as well as many minor species of herbs that enriched our diet and provided health benefits. One result of our modernization of food production has been the loss of this diversity. When I attended medical school almost 30 years ago, I was taught that you get all the vitamins you need by eating the basic four food groups. Today, we know that is not true and that there is a great deal of evidence suggesting that four basic vitamins including multivitamins with folic acid, vitamin E, vitamin C and calcium can benefit all Americans by reducing the risk of chronic diseases.

Also in 2002, *The Journal of the American Medical Association* published a study titled "Vitamins for Chronic Disease Prevention in Adults" that reviewed 30 years of medical research into chronic diseases and vitamins. It was clear to these Harvard University study authors, K.M. Fairfield and R.H. Fletcher, that vitamin and mineral deficits in our diets put us at risk for cancer, heart disease, and a range of other health problems. "All adults should take one multivitamin daily," was their conclusion.

By 2004, the Council for Responsible Nutrition in Washington, D.C., was issuing statements urging consumers to make regular multi-vitamin use a foundation for the protection of good health and the prevention of disease. In particular, the group cited vitamin supplements as bestowing these health benefits: a strengthened immune system, protection against cataracts, improved cognitive function, and building and maintaining strong bones.

Consumer confidence in the idea that our diets can satisfy all of our nutritional needs has plummeted as scientific evidence for the diet deficit accumulates. Surveys conducted in 1994 by the public opinion firm Multi-Sponsor Surveys of Princeton, N.J. found 70 percent of all women in the U.S. believed their diets were adequate for vitamin and mineral intake; but by the year 2000, that confidence percentage was down to just 46 percent of those surveyed.

The fact that only one-third of us regularly use supplements when two-thirds of us are aware of the need to be using them demonstrates the existence of a gap that can only be overcome with proper nutritional education. With all this evidence that our diets alone are no longer sufficient to give us the vitamins and minerals our bodies need, how can we afford NOT to use supplementation to help make up the diet deficit? Your health and the well-being of those you love and who depend upon you may hinge on your answer to this question.

Vitamin Development History

At this point you may be wondering what exactly a vitamin is and how we initially became aware of how important they are to our health. A concise answer to the first part of that question is that vitamins are organic micro-nutrients essential to normal human metabolism. Unlike fats, carbohydrates, and some proteins, vitamins are not metabolized to provide energy. Most are not manufactured by the body but are present in minute quantities in natural foodstuffs. Each of these naturally occurring organic compounds performs a specific vital function and is required by the body for disease prevention and good health.

The known vitamins are divided into four fat-soluble types (A, D, E, and K) and nine water-soluble types (eight B vitamins and vitamin C). The fat-soluble vitamins can be stored in the body and do not need to be ingested every day. Because the fat-soluble vitamins are not eliminated from the body through the urine, ingesting too much of them can create toxicities. The water-soluble vitamins are more easily eliminated and can be taken in larger amounts without much danger of toxicity. Vitamin C and the eight B vitamins (except for vitamin B12 and folic acid) are water soluble. They cannot be stored and must be consumed frequently for optimal health.

As an initial convention, vitamins were given letters to go with their chemically defined names. Not many people may know about the form of vitamin E d-alpha tocopheryl succinate, but most people know what "vitamin E" is and how it can be used. Some nutritional factors were originally given "B" names but turned out not to act as vitamins at all. You may not have heard of vitamins B4, 7, 8, 9, 10, and 11, which were ultimately rejected as vitamin factors.

Although our knowledge and awareness of vitamins as important nutrients came about relatively recently, most of the ancient healing traditions dating back 5,000 years demonstrated some recognition that certain herbs and vegetables contained an invisible substance with an energy or life force that could reverse serious health conditions.

In both ancient Egypt and Greece, for instance, it was known that night blindness could often be successfully treated with carrots. Today we know this old remedy works because of the naturally occurring vitamin A found in that vegetable. Whether by common sense, by the power of observation, or by intuition alone, these ancient cultures understood the principle that a life force within the foods of nature could maintain human health and even restore it.

Our understanding of this principle took a quantum leap forward in 1747, when a Scottish naval surgeon, James Lind, discovered that an unknown substance in lemons, limes, and several other fruits and vegetables prevented scurvy, which was a serious problem for sailors of that period. This nutrient would eventually be identified as vitamin C.

Between 1650 and 1850, half of all seamen on transoceanic voyages died of scurvy. Back then it was a common and deadly disease, and more British sailors were actually lost to scurvy than to the wars they fought. In 1753, James Lind published his *Treatise on Scurvy*, but because he was ignored for another 40 years, more than 100,000 British sailors died from the disease. Later, his work was recognized and appreciated by the Royal Navy, which eventually required that all ships carry citrus and other foods that contain high levels of vitamin C.

Scurvy is a serious hemorrhagic disease that causes lack of energy, immune deficiency, and spontaneous bleeding, often leading to death. Although those who used citrus fruits or chickpea sprouts to prevent scurvy had no concept of "vitamins" as we do today, they did know that there was something in the citrus fruit or vegetables that prevented scurvy. Because limes traveled well, they were the common choice of sea captains, who distributed them to the sailors and crew. The use of limes by the British Navy and other British commercial shipping companies created the slang term "limeys," referring to British sailors and citizens of the British Isles. It was also discovered that raw potatoes, which contain small amounts of vitamin C, could also prevent scurvy.

In the 1860s Louis Pasteur demonstrated that many diseases were linked to microscopic organisms. Soon after, the concept of infection caused by "germs" became the basis of the Western theory of medicine and disease. Around this time, beriberi and pellagra were believed to be infectious diseases. Beriberi can cause mental dysfunctions, weakness and numbness in the extremities, weakening of the cardiac muscles, and heart failure. Pellagra caused indigestion, skin rashes, loss of memory, hallucinations, and eventually death if not treated with B vitamins. It was later discovered by Dr. William Fletcher and others that consuming whole grains, which are rich in B vitamins, prevented this disorder.

The discoveries of the effects vitamins have upon human health developed further around 1905 when an English doctor, William Fletcher, experimented on asylum inmates in Kuala Lumpur, Malaysia. Beriberi was a nutritional deficiency disease common in the rice cultures of Asia back then. Fletcher believed that special nutrients contained in the husk of the rice could prevent beriberi. Fletcher showed that nearly 25 percent of those who received polished rice (white rice) devoid of B vitamins developed beriberi, while less than 2 percent of the 123 patients who received unpolished rice (brown rice) containing B vitamins developed beriberi. His experiments proved his theory, and this led to the discovery of vitamin B1 (thiamine) and other B vitamins.

In 1912, while working at the famed Lister Institute in London, the 28-year-old Polish-born biochemist Casimir Funk took Fletcher's thinking a few steps further. Funk demonstrated that vitamins were vital for good health. He formulated the hypothesis of vitamin deficiency diseases, which stated that a lack of a particular vitamin could cause illness. He isolated the active substances in the husks of unpolished rice that prevented beriberi, and coined the term "vit-amine," which he defined as important substances in food that are vital for life—*vita* meaning "life" and *amine* from nitrogen compounds found in the thiamine (vitamin B1) isolated from rice husks. (The nitrogen compounds were thought to be similar to amines, but the chemical parallel was later disproved.) However, the name and concept of vitamins captured the public's imagination, and later the "e" was dropped and the term *vitamin* was adopted.

The year 1913, however, marked a significant and simultaneously positive and negative turning point in the history of nutritional sciences, when an influential group of scientists turned their attention to finding and isolating the vitamin factors in food.

Thomas Osborne and Lafayette Mendel conducted experiments at Yale University and determined that butter contained a factor necessary for natural growth and development. This factor became known as fat-soluble vitamin A. Its chemical character was established in 1933, and a fractionated form of it was synthesized in 1947. Other vitamin discoveries soon followed. Cow's milk was found to contain growth-promoting factors, which include the water-soluble multiple vitamin B family: Before the 1930s it was only known as "B" vitamin; now we know it as the "B-complex" family of multiple B vitamins.

In 1928, recognizing nutrition as a newly emerging specialty within the biological sciences, a group of visionary American biochemists and physiologists formed the world's first scientific society focused on nutrition. All of its founding members were actively engaged in teaching and writing textbooks and academic articles defining the new discipline, and their new "Nutrition Society" brought much attention to the use of vitamins.

Named the American Institute of Nutrition, the society's original purpose was to publish a journal containing research reports in the newly emerging field of nutrition. Its charter members comprised the editorial board for the Institute's magazine, *Journal of the American Institute of Nutrition*. The society was opened to other researchers in 1933, and held its first scientific meeting at the Cornell Medical School in 1934. In 1941 it was officially affiliated with the Federation of American Societies for Experimental Biology. Today the society, re-named the American Society for Nutritional Sciences (1996), is the world's oldest and foremost nutritional science society.

In the 1930s, a flurry of scientific discovery demonstrated the biochemical functions of various vitamins and established the body's requirements for them. Since then, forms of vitamins have been widely available in thousands of processed foods produced on a massive commercial scale. These synthetic vitamins are fortified into many of our breads, cereals, pastas, and other grain products, as well as many dairy products, drinks, and desserts. In fact, it is nearly impossible to find any fortified food product that does not contain some form of synthetic vitamins.

Although this early scientific community made many valuable contributions in understanding the role of individual vitamins in health, the process of identifying and isolating vitamins led to an incorrect assumption (now shared for nearly a century by a majority of nutritional scientists) that vitamins are as effective and health-promoting in their isolated state as in their natural whole-food state.

These scientists meant well, but they did not realize that their focus and work would help create a flawed foundation upon which the field of nutritional science is built. They simply lacked the understanding that a vitamin's efficacy depended on its cofactors, which are only present when the vitamin is in its naturally occurring state in whole foods, or in the supplements made from them.

Unfortunately, this generally accepted but incorrect "truth" or paradigm remains the guiding philosophy behind modern health, nutrition, and food-science protocols that focus solely on isolating and repairing *parts* of the whole, without regard to the whole itself.

In spite of the abundance of nutritional knowledge, scientists still lack an ability to observe and understand how nutrients work. Quantum science has provided data demonstrating that multitudes of cofactors exist within and around these vital nutritional structures (vitamins) that are essential to its correct functioning. These microscopic and often invisible factors may be as nutritionally important as the vitamin itself. Even at the most basic level, vitamins and minerals will never perform fully without their cofactors. This is why isolated, manmade chemical supplements do not provide the nutrition the body requires. Sadly, they can also weaken the immune system, potentially fostering an environment for disease, which is why we refer to them as toxic.

Fortunately today more people are embracing a natural lifestyle that includes organic whole foods and naturally occurring whole-food supplements as the best path to health and happiness.

Therapeutic Uses of Vitamins

From the discovery of vitamins in 1911 through the 1950s, nearly all doctors based their diagnoses of vitamin deficiencies on readily observable symptoms, such as the hemorrhaging caused by scurvy or the paralysis caused by beriberi. In this period, researchers laid the foundation for a new way of looking at both natural and synthetic vitamins as medicine or drugs.

In the mid-1940s, Evan V. Shute, a medical doctor from Canada, put Hungarian physiologist and discoverer of vitamin C Szent-Györgyi's ideas about vitamin therapy into practice. Shute and his colleagues used large doses of synthetic vitamin E to treat patients with a variety of cardiovascular diseases. Around the same time, Frederick R. Klenner, MD, of Reidsville, N.C., began treating a variety of viral diseases, including polio, with some limited success using large doses of synthetic vitamin C. In 1952, Abram Hoffer, MD, PhD, started treating schizophrenics with synthetic vitamins C and B3 with some positive results. This was the start of a new way of thinking about vitamins in the same way that we think about drugs today.

As we know, isolated chemically produced supplements such as drugs can work well to prevent or suppress symptoms, but we also know that drugs and vitamins made from synthetics also have toxic side effects. Because they are not "nature-made" or a natural whole-food matrix, the body does not recognize them as useful nutritional building blocks. Furthermore, because of their synthetic nature, the body views them as foreign substances, and as such launches an immune response against them. This immune response does not necessarily prevent the synthetic vitamin from alleviating symptoms and giving the impression that healing has occurred. In fact, the reverse is true: When the body is flooded with synthetic substances, it not only loses its receptivity to them, but it also must manage the stress caused by the immune response. This is why there is little success in using synthetic vitamins as part of a long-term treatment program.

The elimination of symptoms is rarely an indicator of health. It is common for people to experience recurrences in disease even after successfully addressing the symptoms. Why? Because the root cause of the disease or illness has gone untreated. Health is only possible when the deficiencies that caused the symptoms, and therefore the disease, are addressed.

As we have pointed out, synthetics of any kind are not usable as nutritional building blocks, and therefore are unable to address these deficiencies on the fundamental level and be an aid to good health. Although synthetic vitamins are likely to have fewer side effects than drugs, it is more helpful to see them for what they are: low-dose synthetic drugs that address disease on the peripheral or symptomatic level. This is the primary argument for their lack of effectiveness as health providers.

Vitamins may be used in emergency-care situations, and many health professionals put vitamins in the same category as drugs. This makes sense; synthetic vitamins *are* isolated man-made chemical compounds and therefore are similar to drugs. Truly naturally occurring vitamins are not at all like synthetic vitamins, and as such are not in the same category as drugs. Naturally occurring vitamins are derived solely from food and medicinal sources such as fruits, vegetables, or botanicals. Synthetic vitamins, on the other hand, are made in laboratories by chemical processes usually from base chemical sources.

As the nature-made molecular structure of naturally occurring vitamins is undisturbed by the manufacturing process and their delicate matrix of cofactors maintained, they are highly usable and effective as nutritional building blocks for the elimination of disease-causing deficiencies and the creation of health.

The Process of Creating Synthetic Vitamin Supplements vs. Naturally Occurring Supplements

Synthetic vitamins, like pharmaceutical drugs, are made entirely in laboratories or manufacturing facilities through a series of chemical manipulations. These proprietary and patented formulations, which may easily require several chemicals and more than a dozen steps, are designed to duplicate the molecular structure of the desired isolated vitamin compound. The specific formulas are not public knowledge; the main point of this brief illustration is that synthetic vitamins are created entirely through chemistry.

Pharmaceutical companies are adept at making various chemical compounds for drugs, and they know how to manipulate chemicals to create specific chemical compounds. Although the original base materials used to make synthetic vitamins may be considered by some to be "natural" or "organic," they are rarely if ever found in synthetic vitamins. Even worse, they may have proven toxicity, as in the case of coal tar and other petrochemicals.

Let's use synthetic vitamin B1 as an example. Starting with a base material such as coal tar, a widely used foundational substance, chemists may add hydrochloric acid or another chemical to create a precipitate—the resulting material when combining two reactive compounds. The formulation, which may include many additional steps including fermentation or some other proprietary or patented process that could involve the use of chemicals and specialized chemical processes, and various heat and cooling reactions, continues, until a copy of the final isolated chemical compound, vitamin B1, is achieved. The final "vitamin" substance is then dried and tested for chemical "purity" and then shipped to distributors or manufacturers who use this synthetic vitamin material in the final manufacturing of their supplement products.

In terms of creating a final product, manufacturers may "contain" the chemical "vitamin" material in a variety of ways: They can utilize any number of excipients, or binders, both toxic and nontoxic, to create tablets; a process of tableting without any excipients at all; or use capsules made of gelatin—an animal product generally formulated from beef and pork hides and byproducts—or, ideally, use vegetable sources such as cellulose (Vegecaps).

The process of creating a naturally occurring vitamin B1 supplement is markedly different. First, the food or botanical containing the desired vitamin or nutrient, such as wheat germ or rice germ, is harvested and cleaned. The food item may then be placed in a large vat where it is mixed with purified water and then filtered to create an extract. The filtration process is used to remove cellulose and fiber, the solid and indigestible non-nutrient parts of the food or botanical. It is important to note that although cellulose and fiber do not contain nutrients in and of themselves, they are exceptionally valuable because of their ability to sweep and cleanse the intestinal tract and promote healthy elimination of the bowels. A healthy diet and sound nutrition plan contain good amounts of fiber on a daily basis. However, when considering a concentrated food supplement with naturally occurring nutrients, the fiber is removed so that the nutrients are absorbed more quickly and efficiently. An example in the world of food is eating broccoli for vitamin A (and other valuable nutrients) and fiber, but drinking some vegetable juice or taking a whole-food based supplement for additional vitamin A.

The resulting post-filtration extract of the food source contains the full spectrum of nutrients and synergistic cofactors as the original food. This extract is then dried, typically at low temperatures and by natural processes rather than freezing or with carbon dioxide or other chemicals, or at high temperatures. Once the extract is dried and tested, it is ready for packaging. In the case of naturally occurring supplements, manufacturers generally prefer using a vegetarian gel cap made from plant cellulose or a tablet made without artificial excipients such as magnesium stearate or other artificial binders or lubricants.

As you can see from this explanation, synthetic vitamin supplements are foundationally and significantly different from naturally occurring vitamin supplements. Synthetic vitamins are pure chemical compounds that have never been alive within a whole food or botanical as created by nature. In their crystalline chemical form synthetic "vitamins" may have a shelf life of thousands of years and are quite stable, just like synthetic drug compounds. In reality, there is nothing truly natural about them.

The Discovery of DNA

Deoxyribonucleic acid (DNA), which contains the biological blueprint of the human body, was discovered in 1944. A year later, Linus Pauling, PhD, developed the concept of "molecular disease" and laid the foundation for modern molecular biology. His ideas set the stage for the use of megadoses of synthetic vitamins. Dr. Pauling became an avid proponent of vitamin use, especially of large doses of synthetic vitamin C.

Another milestone occurred late in 1954, when Denham Harman, MD, PhD, and professor emeritus at the University of Nebraska Medical School, conceived the free-radical theory of aging and the way antioxidants (such as vitamins C and E) can neutralize free radicals and extend life. Harman's idea was simple: free radicals, which are molecules with an unbalanced pair of electrons, react with and damage DNA and other cell components. Harman realized that antioxidant nutrients, such as vitamins C and E, could neutralize these free radicals by combining with them and then chemically neutralizing them, thereby helping the body to eliminate them. Today vitamins like C and E are known to have powerful, active antioxidant qualities when in their complete form.

In 1956 Roger Williams, PhD, published his concept of biochemical and nutritional individuality. Based on extensive anatomical, genetic, and biochemical data, Williams argued that people vary widely in their individual nutritional requirements. He saw the Minimum Daily Requirements (MDRs) and Recommended Dietary Allowances (RDAs) as attempts to create statistical norms of intake when no norms could really be possible. The only reasonable approach, Williams explained, was to strive for optimal nutrition. Dr. Linus Pauling agreed with these ideas and in 1968 described the theoretical foundation for nutritional medicine. Pauling put molecular biology into understandable terms for the lay person. In his concept of "orthomolecular" medicine, Pauling recommended that people use substances (including synthetic nutrients and vitamins) that he considered "normal" to biochemistry.

It is important to note that chemically derived nutrients activate biochemical stimuli, which at first gave the scientific community the impression that these substances were building health. What they were not aware of is that wars were waging between the immune system and these chemical substances, causing an overall deterioration of health.

Since 1955, ongoing research into the functions of whole-food vitamins has shown that they not only help to prevent deficiency diseases, but are also valuable for their medicinal qualities. With naturally occurring whole-food supplements, health is and will be the final result.

Synthetic vitamins, like pharmaceutical drugs, can initially affect positive changes in body chemistry. For example, niacin (B-3) has been shown to be effective in lowering blood cholesterol levels. However, when using any synthetic vitamin or pharmaceutical drug, you are also subscribing to its inherent toxicities as well as its toxic side effects. As an important side note, using chemical supplementation to address symptoms of a disease is simply bad medicine. Symptoms must be addressed on a more fundamental level through dietary and lifestyle changes for any long-term corrective success.

Synthetic nutrient supplements are generally less powerful than pharmaceutical-grade substances, but they all have negative impacts. Promoters of pharmaceutical-grade supplements claim that they are better for you, but in fact, they deteriorate health at the same or greater rate than the average chemically formulated varieties.

Controversial Definitions Emerge

As long ago as the 1930s, a divergence of opinion developed regarding the true definition of a vitamin. Some health professionals defined a vitamin as a naturally occurring complex matrix found only in real foods and botanicals. This definition contrasted with that of chemists and scientists who were synthesizing fractions of vitamin compounds. They defined vitamins as isolated synthetic chemical compounds that resembled certain parts of those naturally occurring vitamin matrices.

A few notable proponents of natural foods and medicine fought against using the synthetic vitamins that the big pharmaceutical companies and their government supporters promoted. One of these early heroes of natural vitamins was Dr. Royal Lee, DDS, a pioneer in natural medicine and one of the first developers of natural vitamin alternatives to the synthetic vitamins of the time.

Dr. Lee was raised on a farm near Dodgeville, Wisconsin; his interest in science and nutrition began at the local elementary school. At age 12, he compiled a notebook of definitions on biochemistry and nutrition and began collecting books on these subjects. Dr. Lee graduated in 1924 from Marquette University Dental School in Wisconsin, where he became primarily interested in the importance of nutrition. A paper he prepared in 1923 outlined the relationship of vitamin deficiency to tooth decay and showed the necessity of vitamins in the diet. Later, Dr. Lee heroically invested time and other resources in battling those that supported synthetic nutrients and synthetic vitamin fortification of foods. Dr. Lee clearly saw the dangers of establishing the use of synthetic vitamins in our food systems. He is still remembered for his efforts to preserve our traditions of natural medicine and for his courage and contributions.

The controversy over the definition of a proper vitamin remains today. It centers on whether a manmade synthetic chemical compound can be defined as a vitamin at all, or whether a real vitamin can be only a naturally occurring matrix found in nature.

Interestingly, the chemists' definition seems to have prevailed in time: Most health professionals, natural foods retailers, and the public have accepted the chemists' definition of a vitamin. This is not surprising, as it generally takes years to shift the collective consciousness. Meanwhile, the highly profitable multi-billion-dollar supplement industry invests millions a year to influence and maintain the status quo regarding public opinion.

The chemists' definition of a "vitamin" takes any isolated part of a vitamin, which looks similar to a natural vitamin part, on a molecular level. Chemists generally do not see any difference between a natural or a synthetic vitamin or nutrient because they look similar to them.

As we know, looks can be deceiving, and a natural vitamin is undeniably different from a synthetic one. Complexes found in nature, with their irreplaceable functions, are greatly superior.

There are four elements within a naturally occurring whole-food supplement that are not analyzed by most chemists. They are: hormones, oxygen content, phytochemical levels (compounds that are naturally occurring in living plants), and enzymes—or H.O.P.E., as we refer to them at the Hippocrates Health Institute. Each of these critical components fulfills nutritional and electromagnetic requirements and is essential for the health and proper function of cells. Because they maintain the activity of vitamins and minerals, they are as important as vitamins and minerals, but they are not yet regarded as such by academic scientists today.

Those who understand that a vitamin is actually a naturally occurring and living-food-based matrix found only in foods and botanicals do not agree with the chemists' view of vitamins. Instead, they reject the notion that, because synthetic vitamins look similar at the molecular level to natural vitamins, they are the same. A photo or a plastic model of a plant may look like a plant, but it is not. The difference between a real, living vitamin and a "dead" chemical compound is the difference between life and death.

One reason that many have accepted the chemical view of vitamins is that the notion of "a better life through chemistry" has become a strongly held belief in our society since its introduction in the 1930s. At that time there seemed to be no limit to what chemistry and technology could accomplish, so people became enamored with chemistry, and the distinction between natural and synthetic gradually became blurred. Today, if you ask a chemist the difference between a synthetic vitamin compound and a natural vitamin compound, the chemist will likely tell you that they are the same. However, the chemical form is "dead," derived from chemicals or manipulated materials, whereas the naturally occurring form is "alive," coming from a source created by nature that exudes life. Synthetic chemicals or inorganic materials are never "alive," as they come from lifeless sources.

Can a fractionalized, isolated part of a vitamin be called a real vitamin at all? These are the important questions we will answer, perhaps for the first time, as we explore the controversy that has, behind the scenes, raged between makers of natural and synthetic vitamins for nearly 80 years. In this book we will help you redefine and understand what constitutes a "real" vitamin. (See the following chromatography example.)

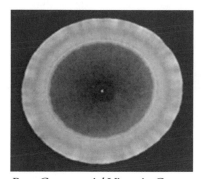

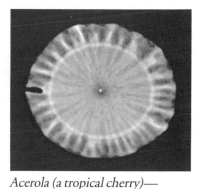

Pure Commercial Vitamin C (Ascorbic Acid).

Typical rings of ascorbic acid but no biologically active ingredients.

Acerola (a tropical cherry)— Natural C.

Jagged border and strong radiations indicate intrinsic factors, vitamins, and enzyme activity.

These diagrams illustrate the intrinsic biological differences between a synthetic vitamin and the inorganic minerals so frequently added, and natural whole-food-based vitamins with their many natural cofactors organized and balanced in nature's laboratory. These chromatograms show that man cannot duplicate what nature creates, even when the chemical analysis is identical.

The nutritional welfare of our people will be inestimably improved as modern nutritional protocols consider this key divergence and the inadequacy of man's efforts to duplicate nature. We are indebted to Dr. Ehrenfried E. Pfeiffer and his staff in their Biochemical Research Laboratory, Spring Valley, New York, for the infinite care and patience in developing these chromatograms.

Globally we have a big job ahead to restore soil quality—even on organic farms—and bring back the nutrients that have been farmed out of our food. It is urgent that we reintroduce organic farming as the primary farming method, as well as the rotation of crops to improve the quality of our soils. It has taken many decades to ruin our soils, and it will take time to revive them and make them healthy again. Meanwhile, the only way we can guarantee getting adequate nutrients is through food supplementation with naturally occurring, non-synthetic vitamins and nutrients, preferably from organic farms that focus on soil conservation.

CHAPTER 2

MISCONCEPTION #2: SYNTHETICS ARE EQUAL TO NATURAL NUTRIENTS

For two decades, we at the Hippocrates Health Institute have conducted an ongoing experiment that is unique in the annals of nutritional science: We have examined through a high-powered microscope the blood of more than 11,000 of our guests who were users of synthetic supplements when they arrived at our institute. We measured the nutrient levels in their bodies before they began our three-week residency program, and after. Specifically, we were interested in the differential between red and white blood cell counts, which are an indication of cell strength (with an increased count) and malabsorption or cell deficiency in the case of decreased counts.

What we discovered has remained constant throughout those two decades: There was little to no absorption and retention of synthetic vitamin nutrients in the more than 11,000 users of pharmaceutical-grade supplements whose blood we drew and tested. Furthermore, we studied leukocytes, with Spectracell technology, to determine which nutrients were being absorbed. The cells in individuals using chemical supplements consistently showed a significant deficiency of nutrients at the beginning of our program compared to the end of the program, highlighting the virtual uselessness of laboratory-created supplements.

Once they enter our three-week program, guests at Hippocrates ingest only a whole-foods organic and raw diet that includes naturally occurring supplements made from whole foods. We offer what is arguably the most nutrient-rich diet of any program in the world. At the end of three weeks we test our guests' blood a second time and compare the before and after results.

What we have measured and documented is the phenomenal ability of the human body to absorb and retain natural nutrients that assist in the process of healing and rejuvenating the immune system. At least 75 percent of people previously taking synthetic nutrients who completed our program showed a dramatic turnaround in the nutrient levels measured in the second round of blood testing. Their nutritional deficiencies had been remedied in that short time frame.

We also noticed that people most saturated with synthetic supplement chemicals exhibited many of the symptoms of drug addiction. I have seen this disturbing phenomenon dozens of times. As they are coming off the synthetics, often the kind that are administered intravenously, they shake and experience tremors. Their eyes roll back in their heads and they sweat profusely. It is a frightening sight. Most of these people were not otherwise ill, but the synthetic supplements were clearly toxic to them.

What we have seen firsthand in a clinical setting has been confirmed by laboratory research that compared natural and synthetic biological effects on the human body. Not only that, but despite what many mainstream chemists may claim—that there is no difference between molecules of synthetic nutrients and the natural nutrients they were designed to mimic—persuasive evidence has accumulated that important differences do exist. These differences in turn affect our absorption of nutrients, and our overall level of health.

One of the more significant studies demonstrating the molecular separation between natural compounds and synthetics was published in 2002 by the *Journal of Chemical Information and Computer Science* in an article titled "Differences Between Drugs, Natural Products, and Molecules From Combinatorial Chemistry." "Natural molecules differ substantially from synthetic ones," wrote the two chemists from Canada who coauthored the study, Miklos Feher and Jonathan Schmidt. They pointed out the ways in which most previous molecular studies had failed to "distinguish natural products and natural product derivatives, molecules that contain both natural and synthetic elements." So these scientists launched a simultaneous and systematic comparison of all three classes of compounds: synthetic drugs, compounds composed of both natural and synthetic materials, and wholly naturally occurring compounds.

"Natural compounds are highly diverse and often provide highly specific biological activities," they concluded. Neither the synthetic nor the partially synthetic molecular compounds could match the natural in the benefits afforded the human body. A key difference was the four-times-higher numbers of "chiral centers" in natural molecules, a term that refers to binding sites that enable molecules to be absorbed by the human body.

Natural molecules contain a greater number of heavy atoms and twice as many oxygen atoms as partial or whole synthetics, and these atoms are also distributed differently in more advantageous ways in those occurring naturally. Photosynthesis and "the pathways leading to different carbohydrates" were identified as being responsible for the higher occurrence of oxygen in natural products. All of these differences contribute to a greater absorption and permeation for natural molecules that makes them much more biologically active, and thus more beneficial to health, than synthetics. The two researchers observed that replacing natural compounds with synthetics relies on "unfavorable modifications" that render synthetics unable to compete with the biological activity of naturally occurring products.

Another reason for differences at the molecular level between natural and synthetic nutrients may have been identified by research conducted by Dr. Gunter Blobel, a cell and molecular biologist at Rockefeller University in New York, who received the 1999 Nobel Prize in Physiology for this work. He found that proteins possess inherent signals or information that determine which cells attract and absorb them and where in the cell the protein belongs.

This finding about proteins opened a doorway for intercellular chemical research that provides us with a principle that has applications for the issue of synthetic and natural nutrients. Nutrients do not simply wander around inside the human body in search of a nutrient-poor cell to colonize. Instead, it is as if nutrients contain addresses and zip codes that enable them to be delivered directly to cells containing the same addresses and zip codes. This is nature's postal system within the body, and synthetic nutrients isolated in laboratories cannot match the simplicity and effectiveness of that system. It is a system that helps to explain why natural nutrients are much more absorbable and bioavailable to us than synthetics.

This point was made more concrete in contrasts that have been made between natural and synthetic vitamin E, an important antioxidant known as the body's lubricant. In a 1998 science article titled "Recent Advances in Oxidative Stress and Antioxidants in Medicine" in *The Journal of Orthomolecular Medicine,* Dr. John Smythies wrote:

> The effective level of vitamin E necessary to protect against heart attacks is between 400–800 mg/day of the natural form. The synthetic form is much less effective. The former consists of a number of stereo-isomers of alpha tocopherol, whereas the latter consists of only one. This difference is important.

Vitamins are biological complexes. They represent multi-step biochemical interactions whose beneficial action depends upon a number of variables within the biological terrain. Correct vitamin activity can only take place when all cofactors and components of the vitamin complex are present and working together synergistically. Vitamins cannot be isolated from their complexes and still perform their specific functions within the cells.

When isolated into artificial chemicalized commercial forms, these purified, isolated, crystalline synthetics act as toxic drugs in the body. Their effect is to compromise the immune system, which can ultimately hasten illness and disease. They are no longer actual vitamins. A vitamin is "a working process consisting of the nutrient, enzymes, coenzymes, antioxidants, and trace mineral activators," as vitamin pioneer Dr. Royal Lee defined it.

Theron Randolph, MD, who in 1965 cofounded the American Academy of Environmental Medicine, wrote four books and more than 300 medical articles and was a leading researcher in the fields of food and chemical allergies, as well as general preventive care. Consider the way he has delineated the difference between natural and synthetic nutrients:

A synthetically derived substance may cause a reaction in a chemically susceptible person when the same material of natural origin is tolerated, despite the two substances having identical chemical structures. The point is illustrated by the frequency of clinical reactions to synthetic vitamins—especially vitamin B1 and [vitamin] C when the [same] naturally occurring vitamins are tolerated" (Tim O'Shea, "Whole Food Vitamins: Ascorbic Acid Is Not Vitamin C" www.whale.to/a/shea1.html).

Synthetic vitamins are actually just fractions of naturally occurring vitamins synthesized in the dextro- and levo-forms (known as right- and left-handed or right- and left-turning molecules) that form geometric mirror images of each other. It may seem strange, but the geometry of nutrient compounds is crucial for the bioavailability of the nutrient. This is also known as the "chirality" of the molecule and relates to the direction in which it turns, specifically to the left or right.

Many organic molecules such as vitamins and other nutritional compounds are chiral and have complex structures that are often asymmetric. Although chirality seems like a subtle difference, it plays an important role in the biological activity of a molecule.

Here is an example of the simplest chiral (right- or left-turning—mirror image) molecule, a carbon with four different atoms bonded to it.

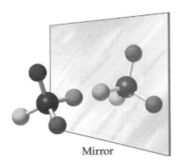

Mirror

The body uses mainly the dextro forms (right-turning forms). Synthetic vitamin compounds have very few of the dextro forms that are present in naturally occurring vitamins, foods, and botanicals. Furthermore, the dextro forms of synthetic nutrients or vitamins are of little use without the associated factors (enzymes, minerals, and other cofactors) that are only present in a whole, natural source of the nutrient or vitamin. Therefore, in order for a vitamin supplement to be effective and fully useful to the body, it must remain in its original and natural state, which contains all the necessary cofactors and dextro-form molecules.

Minerals work through many of the same principles as vitamins. Consider the chromium deficiency that most people in developed countries now experience because that mineral has been leached from our crop soils. In its natural state, chromium contains a glucose tolerance factor (GTF) that helps to protect us against diabetes. But, as the Organic Consumer's Association has pointed out, GTF is not just one factor but a whole family of factors that contribute to health maintenance and prevention. "Almost all chromium products on the market are from chromium picolinate, which is a single isolated compound that is made in the laboratory," wrote a scientist for the OCA in a March 2007 article on its Website titled "Natural or Whole Food Supplements vs. Isolated Chemical Compounds." He pointed out that the compound is missing the crucial glucose tolerance factor, "So it doesn't make sense to take the isolated synthetic chromium supplement. You are not receiving the health benefits. You might as well be throwing your money away."

Our bodies perceive a synthetic supplement just as they would any other foreign chemical: as an invader and a threat to its survival. Our bodies respond by releasing immune-preserving cells such as leukocytes (white blood cells) to combat the enemy invasion. This extra activity distracts these cells from their crucial role of eliminating microbes (viruses and bacteria), spirochetes (such as those that result in Lyme disease), and mutagenic cells (such as those that can result in cancer). With fewer immune-preserving cells at work in our body to combat more deleterious cell activity, there is a greater probability for the emergence of illness and disease.

Synthetics have also been shown to be inferior to natural nutrients at removing toxins from body tissues and organs. Many essential vitamins and minerals are involved in detoxifying us and keeping our immune systems healthy. Vitamin C is one of the more crucial detoxifying agents. When researchers compared pharmaceutical vitamin C to naturally occurring vitamin C based on the ability to remove a common toxin called nitrosamines from the body (nitrosamines are a byproduct of, among other things, cooking processed meats), the synthetics failed to do an adequate job while the natural vitamin C reduced the toxins to much lower levels. That finding was reported by the *Tufts University Health and Nutrition Letter* in 1994. "Vitamins as they appear in nature," the researchers said, "are in complex interrelationships with hundreds, even thousands of other biochemicals within the complex natural food matrix," a synergy which helps to explain why they perform better than synthetics.

You may not want to believe it, but here is the ugly truth about most of the vitamin C sold in the world today: Rather than bolstering your body's defenses against the common cold and other maladies, once in your body most vitamin C sold today becomes tantamount to just another toxin that your organs and immune system must flush out of your system.

Even if the vitamins you take are "natural" ones extracted from food, they will not be effective if they have been removed and isolated from the matrix of complimentary cofactors. Extracting a vitamin from its full-spectrum matrix eliminates the necessary cofactors that assist in the functioning of that nutrient. When you extract and isolate vitamin C (ascorbic acid) from an orange, you are also removing the bioflavonoids that are necessary for vitamin C's complete vitamin activity. It is better to use a full-spectrum concentrate of the whole orange rather than to extract the ascorbic acid or other isolated vitamin C fractions or to take those factors separately.

Nutritionist Dr. Laura Mason-Scarborough, writing for the Holistic Pediatric Association Website, summarized the differences between natural and synthetic vitamin C this way: "What do you get if you purchase a synthesized bottle of vitamin C? You are buying ascorbic acid, a small part of vitamin C, manufactured from refined corn sugar. Ascorbic acid does have strong effects on the body but is more of a drug than a nutrient."

For a complex matrix such as vitamin C to be effective, it has to be used as nature created it. Always use a full-spectrum food source supplement of vitamin C and other supplements to insure that all the naturally occurring nutrient factors are available to your body.

Synthetic vitamin C offers only a fraction of the bioavailability and immune enhancing benefits of naturally occurring sources. If you want a personal demonstration, try this little experiment on yourself the next time you feel you are coming down with a cold.

At the onset of symptoms, take the recommended doses of natural vitamin C extracted directly from Amla berries, an Asian fruit that is a great source for real vitamin C in its most concentrated form. Take daily notes on the effect your dosage has on your symptoms. Keep these notes for future reference because they will be useful in refreshing your memory.

If you continue periodically taking this form of natural vitamin C, you will probably notice that you have fewer colds and less severe symptoms, or no colds at all. But if you are continuing to take the supplement, next time you come down with a cold treat yourself with synthetic vitamin C. Once again, take daily notes on the progression of your symptoms.

Compare your record of experiences with the natural versus synthetic vitamins. People who have conducted this personal experiment invariably report a significant difference. Naturally occurring vitamin C, especially the form extracted from Amla berries, show a remarkable superiority to synthetics.

Natural vs. Synthetic Processes

To package naturally occurring nutrient supplements such as vitamin C from Amla berries, a full-spectrum extract is made by removing the non-nutritive fiber and cellulose from the berries. Then the berries are filtered with water, ground up, and dried at low temperatures to concentrate the nutrients and their cofactors. No high-heat, freezing, or chemical techniques are used in this natural process.

By contrast, synthetics can start in a laboratory with corn sugar or coal tar as a base to create the synthetic nutrients. Ascorbic acid, for instance, can be synthesized from this base using fermentation and chemical manipulations, depending on the manufacturer and its proprietary processes. The ascorbic acid is then marketed as vitamin C.

More Reasons Natural Is Superior

We know that vitamins prevent disease and promote health, but what do we know about the actual quality of the vitamins we ingest?

For more than 70 years we have been consuming synthetic vitamins in our supplements and our fortified foods in the belief that our health is being protected and improved. But what is the real story? Here is the situation we confront with vitamin supplementation and food fortification. There are currently two categories in the family of vitamin and nutritional products with labeled potencies: synthetic and naturally occurring. Nearly all vitamin supplements available today fall into the synthetic category. Some consist of 100-percent synthesized vitamins, and some are combination formulas containing one or more naturally occurring vitamin ingredients combined with synthetic vitamins. Naturally occurring vitamin supplements are composed only of naturally occurring food and botanicals. They contain no synthetic vitamins or nutrients whatsoever.

Synthetic vitamin supplements packaged as tablets, capsules, gelcaps, or powders comprise the majority of vitamin products found in natural-food stores, grocery stores, drug stores, and large retail outlets. Within this category there are certain types and distinctions.

Type 1: In some vitamin supplement products, a natural base is used and then synthetic vitamins or nutrients are added to that natural base. An example of a natural base could be acerola cherry or rosehip, and even a mixture of botanicals. Many vitamin C products that claim to be from acerola or some other fruit or food are usually spiked with synthetic ascorbic acid or ascorbates. Many multiple-vitamin products use a natural base spiked with multiple synthetic vitamins to get their labeled potencies.

Type 2: Some supplements are derived from specially "grown" materials (referred to as "food source" or "whole food" source) such as yeasts and algae. These products typically combine the yeast or algae and create other "mixtures" as a base to which synthetic vitamins are spiked or added. Manufacturers call these supplements "natural" because they are derived from yeast or algae—natural botanicals. However, they are not natural, because synthetic vitamins or nutrients have been added to the product. This is most often not mentioned on the product label and is hidden from consumers, most of whom, ironically, are reading labels to ensure the highest levels of nutrition. Instead, they fall prey to misleading and dishonest labeling information.

The manufacturer of a cultivated base that has been spiked with synthetics nutrients will supply its own as well as other supplement companies with this raw substance. They then use the raw substance to produce and market their own vitamins under different product names. The fact that this raw material contains a cultivated, so-called "natural" base enables the vitamin producers to make the claim on their label that they are derived from "natural sources" and contain the listed potencies from the "food source," referring to the base. As you can now see, this deceptive practice misleads consumers into believing that they have a natural supplement.

Most vitamin companies compete for customers with identical synthetic vitamin products made from compounds produced by the same few drug manufacturers. The vitamin companies differentiate their products with different names and fancy labels, each making claims of "high potency." But the higher the potency of the synthetic vitamin or nutrient, the more likely it is to exhibit drug-like, toxic effects, the stress of which can actually lead to disease.

The majority of vitamin companies also purposely mislead the consumer by taking advantage of loopholes in labeling laws that allow manufacturers to use synthetic vitamins without full disclosure. The truth is that the vitamin potencies for nearly all supplements are derived from synthetic vitamins.

The correct category of vitamin supplements is derived from naturally occurring full-spectrum food and botanical sources. These are truly natural-vitamin potency supplement products and can be identified by their designation "Naturally Occurring" or Naturally Occurring Standard (NOS).

Although vitamins from naturally occurring sources are of a relatively low potency, they are actually much more effective at these lower potencies than synthetic vitamins for the simple reason that the body can easily assimilate their nutrients, and can do so without the toxic side effects of synthetic ingredients.

Just as natural vitamins from food are more effective than synthetic vitamins, so are natural vitamin supplements from whole-food sources. Low-potency vitamins from a full-spectrum, naturally occurring source of the vitamin will produce effective nutrient activity while positively affecting immune function and overall health.

The Vital Role of Bioavailability

Why is it that only nature can create a real vitamin? The differences between vitamins extracted from food and those manufactured by chemical processes is vast, and the distinctions are critically important. Vitamins manufactured in the laboratory come to us without the naturally occurring associated factors and trace substances that ensure a vitamin's bioavailability. If the body can easily digest and absorb nutrients from a food, then they are said to be bioavailable.

Tests on natural versus synthetic vitamins have revealed that synthetic vitamins are less biologically active and bioavailable than natural vitamins. Because our bodies often do not absorb more than 50 percent of the vitamins and minerals we consume, to ingest a product that is already less active than its natural counterpart leaves very little of the original potency available for our use.

It sounds like a simple concept: You are what you digest, or, more to the point, what you assimilate. The digestive system of humans, similar to that of apes, grazing animals, and other herbivores, is complex. The adult alimentary canal measures up to 36 feet; it is long and convoluted. Yet it squeezes into the small space of our abdominal cavity. Many of us assume that we have good and proper digestion and assimilation, and that our bodies can extract nutrients no matter what we eat. This is simply not true, which is why it is important for us to eat wholesome and nutritious foods and maintain high levels of good intestinal flora and other living bacteria that break down our foods completely so that our nutrients can be absorbed.

Furthermore, the human biology has never been able to "digest" synthetic chemicals.

Consider our experience with vitamin E as revealed by numerous science studies. In 1998, for example, researchers with the Linus Pauling Institute at Oregon State University did an experiment in which they gave volunteers 150-milligram doses each of natural and then synthetic vitamin E. Urine tests revealed that the human body prefers natural vitamin E because it retained healthful levels of it while quickly excreting the synthetic vitamin E.

As further confirmation of this finding, Professor Robert Acuff, director of the Center for Nutrition Research at East Tennessee State University, performed an analysis of 30 studies that have been published comparing vitamin E in both its natural and synthetic forms. There was a clear pattern of evidence that natural vitamin E delivers at least twice the health benefits of synthetics because it is much more biologically active and available to the human body.

Even though we may voluntarily or involuntarily (through enriched foods) ingest synthetic chemicals, our digestive systems have not suddenly changed to recognize them as food or nourishment. All the synthetic nutrients in the world are useless, and potentially even dangerous, if they are not digested. The best way to improve digestive absorption of nutrients is to eat good nutrient-rich, living foods and use naturally occurring vitamins and mineral supplements.

"You are what you digest" also means that if your digestion is weak you absorb fewer nutrients from your food than necessary, which can lead to obesity or other imbalances. When enjoying quality foods, the health of your body and all of its systems is strengthened.

As you recall, research with polarized light shows the difference in bioavailability between synthetic and natural vitamins. The beam passing through a natural vitamin always bends to the right due to the direction of its molecular rotation. When passing through a synthetic vitamin, the beam splits in half. Half the light beam bends to the right, while the other half bends to the left. The direction of the molecular rotation makes approximately half the synthetic vitamin impossible to use, which is why there is only 50-percent biological activity or less in synthetic, isolated vitamins. The other 50 percent is of no health benefit—and may even be detrimental—unless the body is able to complete the unusable structures, converting them to forms that can be absorbed and utilized by the body's cells. Chemical supplements lack the factors found in a full-spectrum real vitamin, and are viewed by the body as pollutants rather than as nutrition. What it can convert it uses; the remainder is passed through the system unutilized. The withstanding question is: what do these conversions cost the body, in terms of the nutrients the body must borrow to "complete" the structure; what is the overall stress of this activity?

So what happens to those synthetic vitamins that your body treats as toxins and cannot absorb? The evidence for how much money is being wasted on synthetics that fail the bioavailability test may be found in the Porta Potty business—those portable toilets that have become a fixture on construction sites and at outdoor concerts and other public gatherings. Dr. Joel Wallach, in his book *Rare Earths, Forbidden Cures*, revealed how a friend of his in the Porta Potty business in Grand Rapids, Michigan, would find "literally thousands of multiple vitamin/mineral tablets in the bottom screens when the Porta Potty is pressure-cleaned after a public event."

"How do you know they are multiple vitamin/mineral tablets?" Dr. Wallach asked his friend. "Because the names are still on the coating. One-A-Day, Centrum, etc.," the man replied.

So can a synthesized isolated vitamin fraction made in the laboratory be called a real vitamin? Can it provide you with the nourishment that naturally occurring, whole-food supplements can? The answer is a resounding NO!

Throughout much of the last century, we have been programmed to believe that synthetic chemicals are superior to natural food-source nutritional substances and, therefore, an acceptable substitute. This misleading concept is broadcast mainly by commercial interests that promote this fallacy through sophisticated marketing programs to sell and profit from their inferior "food and nutritional" supplements.

Chemistry has provided us with many benefits, but when it comes to food and nutrition, a better life through chemistry is a fallacy. We are now in the midst of a chemical feast of harmful and polluting chemical preservatives, excipients, colorings, flavorings, additives, and other life-threatening chemicals.

In Western cultures, we have abandoned our history of truly traditional medicine—medicine that has been practiced successfully for thousands of years—and mostly replaced it with technologies dependent on a synthetics belief system. We are now suffering the consequences of this life-threatening decision.

A Synthetics Industry Takeover

It was probably inevitable that the vitamin industry as we know it would be born in the laboratory of a pharmaceutical company. The synthetics belief system that evolved in the first few decades of the 20th century took the "better living through chemistry" faith and the hope that science could improve upon nature and applied it to capturing and imitating a nutrient created by sunshine.

Vitamin C was the logical first choice for synthesizing in a lab because it already had a long history for providing benefits to humankind when consumed in fruits and vegetables. In 1933 a scientist working for the pharmaceutical corporation Hoffman-LaRoche (now known simply as Roche) succeeded at making a synthetic vitamin C by isolating ascorbic acid, which is comparable to the outer skin of an orange. Though ascorbic acid alone lacks all of the nutrient cofactors—those in the body of the orange, in this example—that help to make the vitamin effective, industry chemists rationalized that this aspect of vitamin C was the "active ingredient" that most benefits the human body. Another false magic bullet was born.

This synthetic vitamin creation heralded a pharmaceutical industry attempt at hijacking an idea, that the essential nutrients of plants produced by nature can both maintain and heal the human body. This would be the first of 13 vitamins that would eventually be discovered and synthesized in pharmaceutical laboratories and then mass-produced.

If we examine the short history of synthetic vitamins in more detail, we begin to see some patterns that make it clear why more than 90 percent of vitamins sold today contain synthetic ingredients despite growing doubts about their effectiveness.

1933: Industrial synthesis of vitamin C. Tadeusz Reichstein (winner of the Nobel Prize for Physiology and Medicine in 1950 for work that culminated in the isolation of cortisone) offers Roche a method of synthesizing vitamin C that is effective for mass production. Roche released vitamin C to test markets and sales consistently increased, proving that there was a market for synthetic vitamin C. Because of increasing sales, Roche suspected that vitamin C would be a commercial success and quickly established the process for full-scale production.

1934: Full-scale synthetic vitamin C production at Roche laboratories in New Jersey. This marks the real start of synthetic vitamin manufacturing. At this time, Roche was the only major company producing vitamins; it had no significant competition. Some doctors and other health professionals distributed them, while pharmacies made them available for purchase. Later, the "health food" stores that began proliferating in the 1940s and '50s carried these synthetic vitamins and vitamin formulas.

In the beginning, few people used them. During World War II, however, the government fortified K-rations and the soldiers' foods with synthetic vitamins, which encouraged other companies to fortify their foods in a similar synthetic fashion. The widespread distribution of vitamins began after World War II, when health-food stores and pharmacies began offering lines of synthetic vitamin products, thereby increasing their popularity. By this time, the general public had been educated by corporations on the value of "fortification." This spurred a demand for both fortified foods and supplements—the independent sources of fortification.

1938–1947: Industrial synthesis of vitamin A, vitamin B group, vitamin E, and vitamin K. Industrial synthesis of vitamin A, B1, B2, E, and vitamin K1 is mastered for commercial productions. At the same time, international interest was growing because of the United States' interest in vitamins and its introduction of them into wartime use in fortified foods for the soldiers.

1952: Vitamin products, including supplements derived from synthetic vitamin ingredients, become common as more people became educated about vitamins, and as they became affordable. Many companies that distribute or manufacture health and medicinal products begin buying raw synthetic vitamin materials and manufacturing different brands under many different labels. However, all of these companies were receiving (and continue to receive) their supply of synthetic vitamin materials from only one or two suppliers. At times, companies purchase higher or lower potencies depending on the supply available, but the public is not informed of the difference. As supplements grew in acceptance it caused the manufacturing price to fall, allowing lower costs to consumers and a wider acceptance of their daily use.

Every aspect of the vitamin industry, from food fortification to vitamin manufacturing to sales and labeling, has been manipulated by a few dozen chemical and pharmaceutical corporations that control the synthetics side of this industry. Does that situation constitute some sort of conspiracy? Maybe. It is certainly not an allegation to be made lightly.

The word *conspiracy*, as applied to the synthetics vitamin industry, was first used in a U.S. Justice Department press release. On May 20, 1999, Assistant U.S. Attorney General Joel Klein announced nearly $1 billion in criminal fines against a cartel of vitamin manufacturers, a cartel he said was headed by the pharmaceutical giant Hoffman-LaRoche and other large drug and chemical manufacturers. He described the industry this way:

> The vitamin cartel is the most pervasive and harmful criminal antitrust conspiracy ever uncovered. The criminal conduct of these companies hurt the pocketbook of virtually every American consumer—anyone who took a vitamin, drank a glass of milk, or had a bowl of cereal: This cartel was truly extraordinary. It lasted almost a decade and involved a highly sophisticated and elaborate conspiracy to control everything about the sale of these products. These companies fixed the price; they allocated sales volumes; they allocated customers; and in the United States they even rigged bids to make absolutely sure that their cartel would work. The conspirators

actually held annual meetings to fix prices and to carve up world markets, as well as frequent follow-up meetings to ensure compliance with their illegal scheme. The enormous effort that went into maintaining this conspiracy reflects the magnitude of the illegal revenues it generated as well as the harm it inflicted on the American economy.

As we will see in the next chapter, food and vitamin companies also work together to promote "more chemical supplementation" and "fortification is better" messages when, as we now know, the human body was not designed to respond favorably to synthetic substances.

CHAPTER 3

MISCONCEPTION #3: VITAMIN SCIENCE RESULTS ARE RELIABLE

You may have seen the screaming newspaper headlines that appeared throughout the Western world on February 28, 2007:

"Vitamins Could Shorten Lifespans"

"Supplements Raise Death Rate"

"Another Knock Against Antioxidants"

What the headlines trumpeted was a "meta-analysis" published in the *Journal of the American Medical Association* (JAMA) that purported to show how the consumption of vitamins A, E, C, and beta-carotene—the "antioxidant" group of nutrients—may "significantly increase mortality" among supplement users, "significantly" being defined here as a 5-percent overall increase in the risk of death.

Join the crowd if you found these newspaper articles and the study that spawned them to be confusing and perhaps contradictory. Meta-analysis is a statistical technique that takes the results of many similar studies and gives a summary that is intended to show the weight of evidence. In theory, such an approach to a vast volume of data can be useful and revealing. But in practice this particular treatment of supplement experiments suffered from multiple layers of bias and flawed assumptions.

Out of 16,111 previously published science studies on the health benefits of antioxidants available for inclusion, the authors of this meta-analysis selected only 68 for their statistical comparison, a selection process that was based solely on their judgment. At every step of this process the potential existed for experimenter bias to play a role in skewing the final results.

"This was a flawed analysis of flawed data, and it does little to help us understand the real health effects of antioxidants," declared Professor Balz Frei, director of the Linus Pauling Institute at Oregon State University, one of the world's leading research institutions concerned with vitamins and health. "Instead of causing harm, the totality of the evidence indicates that antioxidants from foods or supplements have many health benefits, including reduced risk for cardiovascular disease, some types of cancer, eye disease and neurodegenerative disease. In addition, they are a key to an enhanced immune system and resistance to infection" ("Study Citing Antioxidant Vitamin Risks Based on Flawed Methodology").

A second critical examination of the JAMA study, this one by physicians associated with the Alliance for Natural Health in Britain (reported in March 2007 on *www.alliance-natural-health.org*, "Alliance for Natural Health Critiques JAMA Study") made an extremely important point about most science studies that attempt to measure the impact of antioxidants and supplements in general—they use synthetic ingredients! "It was seriously remiss of [the JAMA study authors] not to emphasize that the studies they used to condemn these vitamins were nearly all performed using synthetic forms of the vitamins that behave in the body in remarkably different ways to the natural forms," wrote the medical specialists. "In fact, the results tell you absolutely nothing about taking either the natural forms of these supplements, or the effects of taking all these nutrients together, the common way they are taken by most people as multivitamin/mineral supplements."

The primary problem with most supplement studies is their almost total reliance on the "magic bullet" approach to laboratory research that was pioneered and perpetuated by the pharmaceutical industry. It springs from the belief that by merely isolating an "active" molecule or ingredient in any compound, science can create synthetics that mimic the health-giving benefits of the natural sources of those compounds. That approach not only assumes the synthetic molecules act in the same ways as natural molecules, which we have already shown in this book to be a false assumption, but it also ignores the vital role played by the plant source cofactors, and all of the other nutrients that work together as a team to create synergies to benefit human health.

Professor Jeffrey Blumberg, a nutrition specialist and director of the Antioxidants Laboratory at the Human Nutrition Research Center at Tufts University in Boston, has seen this magic-bullet fallacy at work during his research into vitamin E's beneficial effects in retarding the atherosclerotic plaque that causes heart disease. "It is always possible to question whether the dose or form [natural vs. synthetic] of vitamin E or the duration of the study was adequate to find a beneficial effect," wrote Professor Blumberg in a 2002 paper titled "Unraveling the Conflicting Studies on Vitamin E and Heart Disease." "It is also important to note that, to date, all the clinical trials of vitamin E and heart disease have not included any other antioxidants. Yet it is known that the dietary antioxidants, including vitamins C and E as well as the carotenoids and flavonoids, work together in a synergistic fashion."

Elsewhere, in a 2007 interview with CNN ("No scientific evidence diet supplements work," by Caleb Hellerman), Dr. Blumberg pointed out that we have more than 20,000 different antioxidants in our diet. "There aren't 20,000 pills we can take. One of the reasons that dietary supplements can't replace a healthful diet is because we don't know what's important to put in every pill."

In that same CNN segment about dietary supplements, Dr. Andrew Weil made a related and important point: "There's a compound in broccoli called sulphurophane which has been of interest as a cancer-fighting agent. I have seen bottles in health food stores that have a photo of a bunch of broccoli on the label, and the implication is that this is broccoli in a pill. It's not broccoli in a pill. It's sulphurophane in a pill, and that's one element of an incredibly complex plant that has all sorts of different things in it."

Along similar lines, a 1997 study in *The Journal of Orthomolecular Medicine* titled "Beta-Carotene and Other Carotenoids: Promises, Failures and a New Vision," by J.J. Challem, reviewed other research that had that found beta-carotene supplements might increase the risk of lung cancer among long-term cigarette smokers, and cautioned that the synthetic beta-carotene used in the studies and natural beta-carotene have "significant differences that would suggest different behaviors."

"Researchers ignored the likely roles of other carotenoids in health and the possibility that carotenoids...function synergistically," continued Challem. "The use of a single synthetic carotenoid in clinical studies reflects a single-drug magic-bullet approach, whereas the evidence suggests that nutrients work as a biochemical team."

Still another study article from *The Journal of Orthomolecular Medicine*, this one from 1998 by John Smithies titled "Recent Advances in Oxidative Stress and Antioxidants in Medicine" explained in some detail the process by which antioxidant vitamins can work together as a team to prevent the toxin-free oxygen radicals in our bodies from causing disease: "...these antioxidants act in synergism. When vitamin E...neutralizes a toxic ROS [free oxygen radicals], it itself is oxidized." It then needs to be changed back into vitamin E to tackle additional ROS—which is done by vitamin C or glutathione, "which in turn become oxidized. The oxidized vitamin C is converted back to the protective form by NADH, a complex that contains vitamin B3."

Study papers presented in the *American Journal of Clinical Nutrition* by Dr. Gladys Block and others have made supporting cases that because antioxidants work together as a team, those clinical trials evaluating the health benefits of supplements that use only one or even two antioxidants are badly designed, and, as a result, programmed to give us deceptive information.

By reducing the health benefits of nutrients down to a study of individual molecules, argues Michael Pollan, author of the best-selling book on food *The Omnivore's Dilemma*, science researchers betray a "nutrient bias" that is a type of scientific reductionism. Such a study bias will mislead us, writes Pollan, because it ignores "complex interactions and contexts, as well as the fact that the whole may be more than, or just different from, the sum of its parts."

In a thoughtful essay for *The New York Times* early in 2007 titled "Unhappy Meals," Pollan elaborated on this theme: "People don't eat nutrients, they eat foods, and foods can behave very differently than the nutrients they contain...as soon as you remove these useful molecules from the context of the whole foods they're found in, as we've done in creating antioxidant supplements, they don't work at all."

Besides the problem arising from testing synthetic rather than natural nutrients on humans, clinical trials using human subjects to gauge the effectiveness of antioxidants in preventing and treating diseases are flawed in a variety of other ways. According to Dr. Block's study paper "Are clinical trials really the answer?" in the *American Journal of Clinical Nutrition*, the following points that cast doubt on the overall importance of many clinical trials can be made:

⊘ Usually people selected for clinical trials are already at high risk for disease because of their unhealthy diets or other lifestyle factors.

⊘ Rarely do these trials test more than one or two nutrients or more than one dose at a time.

⊘ Trial results tell us little about the prevention of long-term chronic diseases.

⊘ Results reveal nothing about whether the nutrients at high doses might, if taken throughout a lifetime, reduce the risk of chronic diseases.

⊘ Nor do clinical trials reveal the effects of various combinations of nutrients acting synergistically to prevent illness and disease.

There is also a problem in how clinical trials rely upon statistics to the exclusion of patient case histories or medical anecdotes, all of which can reveal important patterns in the ways that we absorb and respond to nutrients. Dr. Abram Hoffer made this point in his 1998 article "Playing With Statistics or Lies, Damn Lies and Statistics" in *The Journal of Orthomolecular Medicine* when he described how the double-blind method used in clinical research has never been validated, in the sense that it has never been proven so reliable that "anyone using the same method will come up with the same answer," the way a ruler is used.

Dr. Hoffer continued on to say that those who completely trust in the double-blind method are not always opposed to case histories, but are "violently opposed to anecdotes. They want to extract bits of information using scales rather than histories.... In some modern clinical accounts of therapeutic trials no patient is evident, only statistics," leading some to question "what species of animal was being tested."

With that observation in mind, it is worth noting that our ongoing vitamin research at the Hippocrates Health Institute offers an important contribution to an understanding of why natural nutrients are superior to synthetics, as measured by thousands of personal case histories we have collected from our guests. Our approach amounts to a five-decade-old clinical trial that embraces, not discards, the individual health experiences of supplement users, because these cases present us with meaningful patterns and tell us insightful stories that statistics alone can never duplicate.

We Are Food Fortification Guinea Pigs

Every single one of us who consumes processed food that has been "fortified" or "enriched" with synthetic vitamins and minerals are participants in a vast and poorly monitored science study that has never been formally acknowledged for what it is—a clinical trial without controls that uses millions of unsuspecting people as guinea pigs.

Consider what we now know about folic acid, a synthetic version of which is added to U.S. cereal grain foods under a 1998 mandate from the U.S. Food and Drug Administration. Naturally found in spinach, broccoli, and other dark leafy vegetables, naturally occurring folic acid works closely with vitamin B12 to metabolize amino acids and synthesize proteins in the body and supports healthy functioning of the nervous system, immune system, and brain.

In 2003 the *American Journal of Clinical Nutrition* published a study titled "Effect of food fortification on folic acid intake in the United States" that was the first to measure and reveal how much folic acid ordinary Americans consume as a result of food fortification. Here is how the study's authors, Eoin Quinlivan and Jesse F. Gregory III, summarized their findings: "Typical intakes of folic acid from fortified foods are more than twice the level originally predicted. The effect of this much higher level of fortification must be carefully assessed, especially before calls for higher levels of fortification are considered."

There you have it! With the best of intentions, a synthetic compound, a type of pharmaceutical drug, is being added to our food supply, resulting in people being exposed to twice the levels that anyone planned or predicted, all with unknown consequences for public health. That amounts to an uncontrolled science experiment in which anyone who eats refined flour or cereal is a guinea pig. A folate toxicity warning label should probably be added to every box of cereal or refined flour product sold worldwide.

Such a warning label could be attached as well to every other food product that contains synthetic nutrients. This would constitute thousands of food products. The more someone consumes fortified foods, the more potential for toxicity exists. Someday researchers will need to undertake the task of measuring what synergistic effect dozens of types of extra synthetic nutrients from hundreds of sources are having on the human body.

Functional foods, the grocery industry term that encompasses "fortification" and "enrichment" with synthetic nutrients, dominate our supermarket shelves. Some functional-food products are marketed to "fix" a condition such as high blood pressure, whereas others are marketed to "prevent" health conditions such as those caused by vitamin deficiencies. Hundreds if not thousands of processed food products are being promoted this way as an alternative to popping pills. But if you fortify a junk food, you are still left with little more than glorified junk food.

A few nutritional authorities recognize and voice the concern that functional foods are not a panacea for good health and may even do more harm than good. "Functional foods are about marketing, not health. Fortification permits manufacturers to market foods of dubious nutritional quality as health foods," writes Marion Nestle, a professor of nutrition at New York University, in her book *Food Politics*. "No functional food can ever replace the full range of nutrients and phytochemicals present in fruits, vegetables and whole grains. The problem with nutrient-by-nutrient nutrition science is that it takes the nutrient out of the context of food, the food out of the context of diet and the diet out of the context of lifestyle."

To some extent in the short term, synthetic vitamins and minerals can have a healthy impact on the human body, especially in cases of severe and chronic deficiencies as found in some less developed countries. But in time, with sustained use and contact from multiple sources, we have seen the positive effects of synthetics rapidly diminish and their broken promises backfire.

Take niacin, for example. Fortification of flour, bread, and rice with synthetic niacin has been credited with almost eliminating pellagra, a nutritional deficiency disease, from the U.S. population. Here is how the synthetic "works" to the extent that it appears effective: When the human body senses the synthetic niacin enter it, the body works to "complete" the whole nutrient of B vitamin complex by attaching other missing elements to the synthetic. It does so by tapping available body stores. Our bodies are very intelligent and try to add the necessary minerals and supporting vitamins that will enable niacin to play its role, but the body can only accomplish this by straining its own physical reserves of these essential elements.

So although fortification may work to partially "treat" or prevent a disease, just as many drugs do, it is not a natural solution. It does not replenish body stores of essential nutrients, nor does it rejuvenate the human immune system, which is the source of true healing. Naturally occurring sources of niacin, by contrast, such as germinated wheat, which contains all of the minerals and other supporting nutrients, provide the type of dietary supplementation that sustains health and promotes longevity.

If past is prologue, as the saying goes, then to understand how we got into this situation we must first take note of how a widespread experiment with our food supply and our health came about.

In the 1920s and '30s, many children lived in crowded cities without much sunshine and ate commercially processed foods that were devitalized of their nutrients. It was discovered that adding synthesized vitamin D to the diet could help prevent children from developing the bone disease called rickets. The U.S. government then required that all milk sold commercially contain this fortification. This step was one of the first global governmental interventions injecting synthetics into a nation's food supply. Soon iodine was being added to salt, synthetic vitamins A and D to margarine, and synthetic vitamins B1, B2, and niacin to flours and breads.

Here is how a food fortification technology text, "Vitamin Fortification Technology," by B. Borenstien, published by the National Academy of Sciences, describes a typical process that adds synthetic nutrients: "Puffed and flaked whole cereals must be fortified at a later stage by a spray, dust, or infusion process. Heat-labile vitamins, such as thiamin, are usually sprayed onto toasted cereals as they leave the oven."

Originally, the term *enrichment* was used to refer to the replenishing of nutrients lost during food processing. Later the term *fortification* came about to include nutrients being added that are not naturally present in the food. Both of these designations are now used interchangeably.

Food fortification and enrichment began with the best of intentions: to remedy nutrient deficiencies in the average diet. But it was also motivated by a synthetics belief system that judged laboratory creations to be equal to, or even superior to, the nutrients of nature. Substituting synthetic nutritional values for real ones became a pattern of accepted behavior for both chemists and food manufacturers. Pharmaceutical producers of such fabricated nutrients also pushed the sale of these chemicals to the food industry via government regulation.

When all-white-flour breads were introduced, synthetic B vitamins were added to the bread mixture to compensate for the wheat germ and other vitamin- and mineral-rich parts of the bread flour that had been stripped away. Although this was good for corporations, reducing the expense of commercial production while increasing profits of their food products as a result of longer shelf life, it was bad for the health of the buying public. The developed world's population, in great part, is now overweight as a consequence, and disease rates are escalating as healthcare costs spin out of control.

The creation of white bread, white sugar, refined flour, refined sugar, and other refined and devitalized foods that began in the early 20th century heralded the emergence of devitalized foods and food ingredients with devastating results.

The so-called fortification process introduced by the food industry as a "cure" is further devitalizing our foods with the addition of synthetic nutrients and inorganic and non-organic materials, which are normally understood as minerals from non-plant sources such as rocks, sand, chalk, and shells. When the terms *inorganic* and *non-organic* are applied to substances of a mineral origin—rather than of plant or animal origin—they are referring typically to substances that have not been "alive" or associated with a living material for thousands and in some cases millions of years.

Raw petroleum oil used to make petrochemicals comes from ancient single-celled animals called diatoms, which were once alive but have been dead for millennia. Rocks such as limestone often come from previously living shellfish exoskeletons or other animal parts such as coral or oyster shells that have been dead and denatured for millions of years. Although these materials may have mineral profiles, we view them as nutritionally void and possibly even harmful; humans are not designed to eat and digest rocks. It is proper for humans to obtain calcium and other minerals (as well as vitamins for this matter) from plant foods that we are naturally designed to digest.

As the purpose of this book is to facilitate an understanding of the true nutritional value of the body of foods and supplements, including whole-food supplements, it is necessary to explain the differences in meaning of the words *organic, non-organic,* and *inorganic* as they are understood and applied by the pharmaceutical industry, the natural food industry, and the general food industry. The differences in meaning can be quite significant and cause a great deal of confusion when considering the overall nutritional and health value of any substance. However, with greater understanding you will be in a position to make correct and relevant evaluations of nutritional supplements.

We'll start with the term *organic*. There is a subdivision in the field of chemistry called "organic chemistry." Scientists in this field use the word *organic* when referring to any molecule or compound that contains a "hexane" ring, which is a specific arrangement of carbon and hydrogen atoms. These "organic" compounds may offer no nutritional value, and in some cases be considered deadly. An example of this is gasoline. Gasoline and other petroleum derivatives, for that matter, are considered "organic" according to the principles of organic chemistry because of their molecular structure, but they are obviously neither a source of nutrition nor safe for human consumption.

The problem arises when chemists from the pharmaceutical industry—an industry that uses the same definition of *organic* as the field of chemistry and supplies more than 95 percent of all "nutritional" supplements on the market today—assume that ingredients are safe for human consumption just because they are "organic" by their definition (in other words, contain a hexane ring). Hexane, coal tar, and other poisonous substances are widely used in the production of synthetic supplements today, yet they are considered toxic by the natural foods and nutrition industries. The safety of these materials remains largely unquestioned and untested because the pharmaceutical industry—an all-powerful and extremely influential industry that is intimately and politically connected to the regulatory bodies that govern the safety of their products (the U.S. FDA and their global equivalents, for example)—considers them safe. Unfortunately, millions of people worldwide are consuming these substances, completely unaware of their harmful nature and of the destructive political landscape that allows and supports their use.

In the field of food and nutrition science (which includes wholefood supplementation), the terms *organic* and *non-organic* have significantly different meanings.

The term *organic* as used in the general and natural foods industry has two primary definitions, both having significance as they relate to human health. In general, *organic* refers typically to substances derived from a living or recently living organism such as a plant, botanical, or animal. By this definition, the unprocessed foods we consume—in total—are considered organic. It is important to note here, however, that based on Hippocrates Health Institute's extensive more-than-50-year history and results in helping people reverse serious and life-threatening illnesses, only plant-based foods and plant-based, whole-food supplements are considered nutritionally relevant and effective. Hippocrates has published many volumes on this position; these books are available by contacting us directly. See Appendix C in the back of this book for more information.

The term *organic* also refers to methods by which a food or botanical is grown and processed. The current USDA designation of *organic* is what most people understand and support; this basically refers to foods that are grown and processed without using most conventional pesticides, fertilizers made with synthetic ingredients or sewage sludge, bioengineering, or ionizing radiation. There is also a large component of organic farming that addresses soil quality, which leads to far more nutrient-rich foods and botanicals.

A *non-organic* food, on the other hand, is a plant or botanical that is grown using conventional farming practices, which include the use of pesticides, herbicides, fungicides, and other harmful chemicals. Non-organic foods and botanicals are lacking in overall nutritional value for two primary reasons: The soils in which they are grown are severely depleted in minerals and nutrients due to conventional farming practices, which include the use of synthetic fertilizers and chemicals. Secondly, the toxic chemicals in and on the non-organic foods that we consume must be isolated and removed by the body; meanwhile, these chemicals cause damage to healthy cells and tissues—damage that in time can result in disease.

Additionally, the term *non-organic* may be used in the food industry to mean that a substance is not recently from a living organism such as a plant, botanical, or animal. Using this definition, those in the field of food and nutrition sciences would label substances such as minerals from rocks and gasoline as non-organic. They have no nutritional value and are even considered toxic to the human body, as compared to an organic material like a recently harvested vegetable or botanical. In this text we will use the terms *inorganic* and *non-organic* interchangeably to mean materials or substances that are dead and not recently from a living organism.

Let's also be clear about what we mean by an "organic" mineral. As you recall, we defined *inorganic* or *non-organic* minerals as minerals from non-plant sources such as rocks, sand, chalk, and egg shells. In this text, we will use the term *organic mineral* to mean that the mineral is from a living or recently living food or botanical source, regardless of the farming methodology. Minerals, similar to vitamins, are in every food and whole-food-based supplement we consume. These minerals generally come from the soils in which a food is grown. As a general rule, foods grown in organic soils provide significantly greater amounts of minerals than those grown at conventional farms.

In summary, when it comes to nutrition, inorganic/non-organic (dead), non-food ingredients, including synthetic vitamins and inorganic minerals, are not recognized by the body as nutrition, even though they may have contained "life" in their original form millions of years ago. In fact, overwhelming evidence points to the fact that adding synthetic, inorganic minerals or toxic nutrients to the human body is worse for health in the long term than adding nothing at all.

Buyer beware! Check your product labels carefully to determine if the vitamin and mineral supplements you consume are derived from food. The human body requires real, living, and preferably organically grown foods and whole-food supplements for health.

In the last several decades at Hippocrates, as I earlier indicated, we have observed ongoing noxious conditions caused by synthetic supplements. In every person who consumes these false nutrients, we detect, microscopically, an overall weakening of healthy active and developing cells. This slow but sure poisoning weakens the immune system and eventually erodes mental and nervous system function, resulting in an overall reduction in the individual's well-being and an ongoing, dramatic biological harm of the cells that inherently create all soft and hard tissue.

Another reason for the genesis of fortified foods was the alarming devitalization of farming soils. Following the German agricultural methods of chemist Justus von Leibig in the mid-1800s, American farmers— much later on—found that using NPK (nitrogen, phosphorus, and potassium) made crops look good to the consumer because they were brighter in color. As long as NPK is added to the soil, crops can be produced and sold year after year from the same soil. But the appearance of food crops can be deceiving, because trace minerals vital for human nutrition have become virtually absent from most of these soils and their resulting crops.

Minerals such as zinc, copper, and magnesium are necessary cofactors of vitamin activity, acting as facilitators. Depleted topsoil is one reason why we have both vitamin and mineral deficiency in crops today, as opposed to those grown before the depletion of our original quality topsoil. The uncountable tons of poisonous herbicides and pesticides dumped on crops throughout the years have not helped our soil at all.

Truly vital foods must be grown in healthy soil rich in both minerals and soil-based organisms. Healthy crops naturally resist insects and bad weather. When crops maintain a healthier immune system, their natural anti-insect and anti-disease mechanisms work more efficiently—just as a human who has a strong and healthy immune system is far less likely to develop diseases.

We must encourage authentic global organic and biodynamic farming. Soil must be brought up to fully healthy standards by dramatically increasing its organic matter. When this is accomplished, those foods grown in such soils will again be rich in the full spectrum of nourishment that our bodies require. Each cell, including immune cells, can then function properly to create strong bodily systems and a heightened immunity.

Naturally occurring supplements must also be made from nutritious foods that are full of vitamins, minerals, and trace elements. Nutrition in a bottle unquestionably depends upon the original food source being complete, bioactive (alive), and organic. Equally important for the quality of a supplement is the process by which it is manufactured, the conditions under which it is transported and stored, and the bottle or container in which it is placed. Dried-food sources of nutrients are fine if they have not been heated at temperatures higher than 118 degrees Fahrenheit (42 degrees Celsius) or dehydrated using chemicals or other synthetic substances. The best dried-food sources come from low-temperature vacuum drying rather than high-heat spray drying, which can destroy naturally occurring enzymes and damage the stability of delicate nutrients such as antioxidant vitamins like vitamin E and vitamin A.

Does anyone want to eat devitalized food? Of course not. But you might be surprised at the reason why many of our foods were refined and devitalized in the first place.

Modern commercial food producers were obsessed with longer shelf life and ease of handling for the processing, transport, and storage of their products. Longer shelf lives for food saved the producers time and money, but as a consequence it devitalized and devalued our foods.

The devitalization of foods and food ingredients through the process of administering high heat was accomplished by removing the nutrients that oxidized (decayed) in order to create food products that could last for years instead of weeks. For example, fresh whole-grain wheat bread with the wheat germ removed allowed for a much longer shelf life. This is because the wheat-germ nutrients oxidized faster than the non-nutritive purely white, mostly carbohydrate part. This massive heat processing also creates acrylimides, a well-known cancer agent.

Although natural preservatives and other means of packaging could have been used as an alternative to prolong the shelf life of the wheat bread, it was easier and cheaper to just remove the essential nutrients. After devitalization, the remaining bleached and/or devitalized white flour bread could last for months or years instead of only days or weeks.

Adding insult to injury, the merging food irradiation industry employs its methods on many of our foods, rendering them virtually neutered. Herbs and seasonings have been subjected to this treatment for decades. All of this was great for increasing the profits of the food processors but detrimental to the health of consumers.

The same sad story of devitalization of wheat flour is also what happened to dozens of other foods and food ingredients such as re-fined grains (like corn flour) and other natural foods. One solution to the problem would be to stop fortifying foods or food ingredients with synthetic vitamins or non-organic substances, and to cease devitalizing foods by removing their naturally occurring nutritional factors. But that would be common sense and health sense, not necessarily business sense.

These comments made in a 1940 issue of *The Journal of the American Medical Association* illustrate that we knew, even then, of the dangers posed by denatured foods. "Until all the factors lost in milling are known and it is known that each of the others is adequately supplied by other foods, the logical solution of the problem presented is the resto-ration of the grain embryo [germ] itself to the diet" (Waisman and Elvehjem, "Multiple Deficiencies" http://jn.nutrition.org/cgi/reprint/20/6/519.pdf).

Here is another medical journal reference from the same period, also by Waisman and Elvehjem, this one from the *Journal of the American Dietetic Association*: "I am very familiar with the difficulties involved with the fortification of foods with synthetic vitamins.... Likewise, synthetic vitamins should be used with caution in order to prevent the development of deficiencies more serious than the deficiency we set out to control." In other words, biochemist Conrad Elvehjem is telling us that synthetic vitamins may not combat any vitamin deficiencies and may actually cause additional health problems.

Also back in 1941, medical and nutritional institutions knew that devitalizing foods such as grain flours and then fortifying them with single synthetic vitamins was detrimental to health. Once again, here is an entry from the *Journal of the American Medical Association*: "The Nutrition Committee of the National Health and Medical Research Council considered the proposal fully but decided that the addition of synthetic vitamin B1 alone to white flour involves a wrong principle" ("Proposed Fortification of White Flour with Synthetic Thiamine" Our Regular Correspondent. http://jama.ama-assn.org/cgi/reprint/116/9/882.pdf).

Despite such findings, the marketing of fractionated crystalline synthetic vitamins has been so universally adopted today that most nutritionists and doctors are unaware that an essential "life force" is missing from these suspect products. At the same time, vitamin manufacturers compete for customers with identical products because they all buy their synthetic vitamins from the same few drug companies. To differentiate their products, companies often make marketing claims of "high potency." But what does that really mean? Quite simply, the higher the potency, the more drug-like effects that occur in our bodies, and, as a result, the more we become guinea pigs in this uncontrolled but money-making public experiment.

CHAPTER 4

MISCONCEPTION #4: YOU CAN TRUST THE "NATURAL" LABEL

What is the prevailing public attitude toward the use of natural vitamins?

"Supplements have come to be seen as a tonic to the influence of drug companies, in much the same way that Apple computers are seen by their ardent users as a shield against the evil empire of Microsoft," wrote Dan Hurley in his book about the supplements industry, *Natural Causes.* "Supplements are the anti-drug, representing everything that drugs are not. Where drugs are artificial, supplements are natural."

Hurley neglected to point out how misguided that perspective turns out to be, given that practically all vitamins and supplements are synthetic, not natural, and made by the very pharmaceutical and chemical corporations that are behind the "better living through chemistry" belief system.

It is probably true that health-conscious people want to believe supplements are free of the pharmaceutical drug stigma. For most of us, *natural* equals *healthful.* We want to believe that, when we see the word *natural* on a label, it actually means something that is verifiable and truthful.

In an ideal world our use of the word *natural* would mean just exactly that: undiluted and direct from nature. Reality tells a different story. As the National Consumers League pointed out in a 2002 study of labels, "products with the 'natural' labeling are not required by law to contain only natural ingredients."

Worldwide, there is no official government-regulated definition for the term *natural* that represents a standard used by the natural products industry. In the United States, the Food and Drug Administration refers to natural ingredients as "ingredients extracted directly from plants or animal products, as opposed to being produced synthetically." But that definition overlooks the loophole that allows chemical additives to be routinely mixed with "natural" ingredients and marketed to the public as wholly natural products.

It is laudable to try to set a realistic legal definition for *natural*, but another problem is that the FDA's system of standards for vitamins has not been based on nature. This system, known as the Recommended Daily Allowance (RDA), or what has now been updated to Daily Values (DVs) and Recommended Daily Intakes (RDIs), relates to the amount of vitamins it is estimated that we require daily for maintaining health. It is based on the assumed nutrient value of synthetic supplements.

The RDAs, DVs, or other "standards" that are generally accepted and used by most agencies and institutions of government and industry were originally established through animal testing using synthetic vitamins—supplements that were not totally digestible and severely lacked nutritional value.

For some consumers the word *natural* is also synonymous with *organic*. Do not be fooled. "This is part of a gigantic hoax being foisted on the public," says Ronnie Cummins, director of the Organic Consumers Association based in Minnesota. "Vitamin makers do not want the public to know that not only are their vitamins not organic, but they're spiking most of them with synthetic vitamins and minerals."

Even when a synthetics manufacturer uses natural plant-derived ingredients in supplements, whether in part or whole, these are usually non-organic plant sources that have been exposed to the full range of noxious chemicals from pesticides to herbicides. There are many other deceptive practices with vitamin labeling that you should be aware of if you want to protect yourself and your loved ones.

On some vitamin labels you may also see the phrase "time release," which implies that the vitamin will be released into your system in such a way as to ensure maximum absorption by your body. No regulations or regulatory agencies require supplement makers to actually prove their products are time-released as advertised. As a result, many vitamins do not dissolve completely as they make their way through your intestinal tract, staying mostly intact until they end up in sewer systems.

Dosage amounts listed on the label may also be misleading. Actual dosage levels can be different, usually higher rather than lower, to account for the substance disintegrating in time and losing its potency. Using a higher potency of ingredients than labeled, done to extend shelf life, is called "building in an overage." Improper storage with exposure to heat, light, air, or moisture accelerates the disintegration rate of all vitamins and supplements. So when you take supplements, especially if you are eating any "fortified" foods, bear in mind that this combination may be contaminating your body with toxic levels of synthetics.

Additives That Masquerade Under "Natural"

Most consumers seem to assume that additives in their supplements are safe and effective, having been proven so by impartial testing facilities and then identified on product labels. That is a dangerous assumption. Chemical additives are not guaranteed to be any less toxic than any other synthetically made chemical compound. When synthetic nutrients or synthetic additive materials are used, we must recognize that, by virtue of them being unnatural and foreign to the human body, they may pose unpredictable risks to your health.

Excipients are additives used in creating tablets or capsules of nutritional supplements. They hold the ingredients of a tablet together during its mechanical creation. This general category of additives might also include natural, artificial, and synthetic colorings, as well as coatings and flavorings. These can be benign or toxic depending on whether they are synthetic or naturally occurring, and also depending upon the sensitivity and reaction of the persons who ingest them.

Most food supplements are packaged in a delivery system that includes tablets or capsules, though they sometimes appear in liquid forms. These can be hard- or soft-shell gelatin capsules, vegetable capsules, or coated or uncoated tablets. The manufacturer puts a powdered form of the vitamin or nutrient into the capsule using encapsulation machinery. The powdered material must flow properly into the capsule and the capsule must be filled completely. Natural excipients like cellulose, rice powder, or other materials may be used to accomplish this.

With regard to capsules, most people prefer vegetable caps made of vegetable gelatin from seaweeds to capsules that use animal gelatin. Animal gelatin is typically made from tallow, animal bone, bone marrow, or animal tissue scraps, including diseased organs and tumors. A frightening aspect of any animal product is the potential for traces of animal feed toxins and hormones, or animal pathogens such as those causing mad cow and other diseases.

The Health Impact of Synthetic Additives

Certain people may be allergic to excipients or additives, so it is important to examine product labels carefully to know that what you are getting is safe. It is best to choose a tablet that is either uncoated or coated with a natural food source. Many chemical companies are actually using coatings derived from beetles, purchased from insect farms in Asia. So you are ingesting bug parts without being told.

Numerous vitamin brands are processed at high temperatures and contain petroleum-derived chemical solvents such as ethyl cellulose, or have been coated with methylene chloride, a carcinogen. Dr. Zoltan P. Rona, the Canadian physician who is medical editor of *The Encyclopedia of Natural Healing*, relates how some people may experience allergic reactions to these additives, with symptoms ranging from fatigue and memory loss to depression and insomnia. "Although most healthy people will have no obvious side effects from ingesting small amounts of toxins found in cheap [synthetic] vitamins, the long-term consequences of continuous daily intakes are potentially dangerous. Over 7 percent of the population displays sensitivity to these chemicals."

Synthetic dyes and flavorings are often used in vitamins marketed to children; those additives pose particular dangers to a child's development and mental health. Two artificial colorings to beware of are Red 40 and Yellow 5, but equal vigilance should be paid to the artificial sweeteners used in children's vitamins, such as aspartame and saccharin, along with preservatives like BHA, BHT, and TBHG. Those additives may have obscure chemical names you have never heard of before, but they are names you would do well to enshrine in your memory. Here is why.

In 1999 a report was prepared by the Center for Science in the Public Interest that reviewed 23 controlled peer-reviewed science studies on the effects of food dyes and other additives on children's behavior, particularly in contributing to attention deficit hyperactivity disorder (ADHD). Out of the 23 studies, 17 were revealed to have "found evidence that some children's behavior significantly worsens after they consume artificial colors." Symptoms of ADHD include impulsiveness, restlessness, reduced attentiveness, and loss of concentration. Some surveys have estimated up to 17 percent of school-age kids have the disorder.

The first evidence of a connection between diet and behavior emerged in the 1970s when a California allergist, Benjamin Feingold, discovered that when he took some children off all artificial flavorings and colorings, their behavioral problems diminished. Subsequent controlled studies bore out that connection, and numerous foods, including vitamins marketed to children, were identified as contributing to the mood swings and the development of behavioral disorders.

A specific recommendation of the report by the Center for Science in the Public Interest was that "manufacturers of vitamin supplements popular with children should minimize the use of dyes and other unnecessary additives." This warning and recommendation has been ignored by the synthetics vitamin industry ever since the report's release in 1999, nor is there any evidence that mainstream medicine has awakened to the fact that synthetic chemicals in diet can provoke adverse behaviors, whereas eliminating those synthetics can restore balance to moods and health.

The effects of chemical additives in our supplements can have profound effects in other ways as well. A U.S. Olympic swimmer, Kicker Vencill, was banned from the 2004 Athens Olympics because he tested positive for a steroid precursor he had unknowingly ingested from vitamins. He sued the U.S. manufacturer in 2005 for contaminating its product and won a large monetary judgment in a California court. The International Olympic Committee did random tests of 240 common supplements and discovered that one-fifth contained synthetic substances that the IOC had banned. None of those substances, of course, showed up on the labels.

Synthetic vitamins should really be treated as pharmaceutical drugs because both categories of synthetics are refined, high-potency chemicals that can only be accurately measured in milligrams. But even the act of measuring a synthetic vitamin compound tells us little or nothing about real vitamin activity or real nutrition and the effects within our bodies. Only naturally occurring nutrients derived directly from plant-based sources can inform us in a way that provides accurate standards of measure.

We often hear suggestions that we should take thousands of milligrams of synthetic vitamin C or E or A by intravenous means. This action is not only challenging to your immune cells but also sends your body into a state of confusion. A noxious biochemical chain reaction begins, with the body working to eliminate these toxins so none of the false nutrients enter the system. When someone experiences dangerous side effects from synthetic vitamin consumption, it is because the chemicals cannot be utilized or metabolized and build up in the body as toxins.

On the other hand, complete food-based vitamins C, E, and A have lower milligram levels, yet the body and blood cells can easily absorb and use them, resulting in an overall increase in health.

Some synthetic vitamins are made from coal tar. This base material, typically a crystalline yellow coal tar derived from fossil fuel sources, is not only used as a base to make many synthetic vitamins, but also as a host for other synthetic compounds including colorings, paints, and other chemical materials used as ingredients. Coal tar is widely used in both the food and cosmetic industries and at certain concentrations can be carcinogenic.

Common Excipients and Additives Found in Food Supplements

⊘ *Fillers* are used to increase the volume of material in a tablet or capsule to create standard-size tablets and full capsules. Common non-food fillers like talc (a known carcinogen) or silicon may cause problems with digestion and absorption. Food-grade fillers include cornstarch, lactose, cellulose, sorbitol, and calcium phosphate.

⊘ *Binders* are various compounds used to bind the components within the tablets together and increase the hardness of the tablet. Binders are made from lecithin, honey, sorbitol, gum arabic, and cellulose.

⊘ *Disintegrants* are added to many supplements to aid in the disintegration of the tablet within the gastrointestinal tract. They cause the tablet to swell and break apart. Some disintegrants have been associated with asthma attacks, rashes, and allergies. In addition, they may contribute to plaque and hardening of the arteries.

⊘ *Lubricants* and flow agents aid in the release of tablets from molds and dyes, and ensure unrestrained movement of materials through the tableting machinery to make the manufacturing process smoother. Magnesium stearate, calcium stearate, and stearic acid may be used to increase the time tablets take to dissolve. Other common flow agents are vegetable stearin and silica. These unnatural materials, like lubricants, have been known to cause indigestion and other health problems.

⊘ *Flavoring agents:* Sweeteners commonly found in supplements are sucrose, fructose, maltodextrin, sorbitol, and maltose. Sweeteners are used in liquid, powdered, chewable, or sublingual supplements. Artificial or natural flavoring may also be added. All of these sweeteners and flavorings are chemically synthesized and are extremely harmful due to these sweeteners fueling viruses, bacteria, and cancers.

⊘ *Coloring agents* are generally added for marketing purposes, specifically to improve the appearance of a supplement. Some are derived from natural sources like beets, carrots, or chlorophyll, but most are toxic synthetics that negatively impact one's health. Many of these dyes, such as the red variety, have a direct link to cancer development.

⊘ *Coating materials* are used to increase shelf life, protect from moisture, and mask unpleasant odors and flavors. Coating also aids in swallowing a tablet and helps to prevent tablets from breaking apart. Coating materials, which are commonly listed on labels as pharmaceutical glaze, confectioners glaze, or natural glaze, are actually shellacs that are difficult to digest, and those derived from petrochemicals are known carcinogens. As stated before, shellacs are often made from the wings of beetles, and natural vegetable coatings are often derived from corn or palm trees.

⊘ *Preservatives.* Some companies use health-promoting natural preservatives such as natural vitamin C or E. Others may use synthetic vitamins or synthetics like nonorganic forms of sulphur or selenium.

All chemical additives, preservatives, and other inorganic or toxic chemicals added to foods are always there for the convenience of the processor or maker of the finished product—not the consumer. The product manufacturer wants the product to have a long shelf life, to look nice, smell nice, and be attractive to you, and the manufacturer usually wants to do this in the least expensive and quickest way possible for maximum profit. Only when consumers demand that the manufacturer eliminate toxic chemicals from the product by voting with their wallet do manufacturers take notice.

Be on the lookout for the synthetic additives listed here:

⊘ *Hydroxypropyl methylcellulose* is a vegetable gum used as a disintegrant and emulsifier in artificial tear solutions. It is resistant to bacterial decomposition. At this time there is no known toxicity.

⊘ *Cellulose starch* made from plant material is used as filler, binder, and disintegrant. Starches processed from corn contain free glutamic acid (MSG). Monosodium glutamate (MSG) was once banned by the U.S. government because of its cancer-causing effects but was reintroduced after serious opposition from the food industry in response to declining sales.

⊘ *Croscarmellose sodium* is a disintegrant derived from vegetable fiber. This excipient is processed with large quantities of chemicals and may contain chemical residues.

⊘ *Sodium starch glycolate* is a disintegrant made from potatoes, maize (corn), wheat, rice, or tapioca starches. It is used in tablets containing insoluble ingredients such as magnesium stearate to help them break apart.

⊘ *Silicon dioxide*, also known as silica, is a transparent, tasteless powder that is practically insoluble in water and known to cause hardening of the arteries. It is the main component of beach sand and is used as an absorbent and flow agent in supplements. It is also used in ceramics, and scouring or grinding compounds.

⊘ *Hydroxypropyl cellulose* is a vegetable gum used in pharmaceutical manufacturing applications and as a disintegrant and emulsifier in supplements. Cellulose in small quantities is generally not known to cause ill effects. However, this excipient may be processed with large quantities of chemicals and therefore may contain chemical residues.

⊘ *Red 40 Lake* is an insoluble pigment used in food, drug, and cosmetics applications. The National Cancer Institute reported that p-credine, a chemical used in the preparation of Red No. 40, was carcinogenic in animals.

- *Polyethylene glycol 3350* is used as an emulsifier, binder, and surfactant (lowers surface tension of materials to help make a dry tablet or disperse a liquid product), which improves resistance to moisture and oxidation. Polyethylene is a polymerized ethylene resin and glycol is an alcohol; both can cause coughing and other toxic conditions. Chemicals such as ethylene resin and others that come under the designation of "plastics" may also disrupt the balance of estrogen in the body. Elevated estrogen levels are both a known cause and symptom of certain cancers. Plastics "out-gas," or expel gaseous fumes from their chemical constituents, which is essentially chemical pollution. It is toxic and unhealthy.

- *Magnesium stearate* is a flow agent and surface lubricant from animal or vegetable sources. It is insoluble in water and said to be non-toxic, but it may hinder the absorption of nutrients and may also have other toxic effects because it is normally made with hydrogenated fats.

- *Resins* are used as binders and aid in water resistance. They may be of plant or synthetic origin, and are used in lacquers, varnishes, inks, adhesives, synthetic plastics, and pharmaceuticals. Synthetic forms include polyvinyl, polystyrene, and polyethylene. Most of these resins are like plastics, which out-gas chemical pollutants. Similar to most plastics, resins have some toxic effects, mostly because they are ingested and deposited in tissues throughout the body, creating unknown damage.

- *Dicalcium phosphate* is a mineral complex of calcium and phosphorous commonly used as a tableting aid, filler, or bulking agent. Phosphates can induce the same symptoms as MSG in those who are extremely sensitive to MSG.

- *Polysorbate 80* is a non-ionic surfactant polymer containing oleic acid, palmitic acid, sorbitol, and ethylene oxide. It is made by microbial fermentation and used as an emulsifier, dispersant, or stabilizer in foods, cosmetics, supplements, and pharmaceuticals. Polysorbate 60 and polysorbate 80 may be contaminated with 1,4-dioxane, a carcinogen. Dioxane readily penetrates the skin. Although dioxane can be removed from products easily and economically by vacuum-stripping during the manufacturing process, there is no way to determine which products have undergone this process. Labels are not required to note this information.

◊ *Titanium dioxide* is an inorganic (indigestible) oxidant used as a whitening agent that has no health benefits, and in fact could cause pulmonary irritation, among other negative reactions. It is used in paints, coatings, plastics, paper, inks, fibers, food, and cosmetics. This material is used mainly to improve the aesthetic appeal of products.

◊ *Povidone* (*PVP*) is a synthetic polymer used as a dispersing and suspending medium.

◊ *Pharmaceutical glaze* is shellac used by some manufacturers to coat vitamin tablets. Shellac is insoluble in stomach acid and difficult for the body to assimilate.

Uncovering Off-Label Ingredients

If you really want to find out what ingredients are in your favorite vitamins, Andrew W. Saul, author of *Doctor Yourself*, recommends that you contact the manufacturer and "politely ask for a full disclosure of ALL ingredients and excipients in every nutritional product the company sells." He lists four possible responses you might get, each one revealing something useful.

1. If the company fails to respond, this will tell you a great deal about the reliability of that brand.

2. The manufacturer might dismiss you with a generic letter saying they use "the finest ingredients." Such a response may mean they have something to hide.

3. Should the company simply repeat the language on its ingredients label, their failure to provide full disclosure provides a reason not to buy the product.

4. Reputable companies will provide a prompt and full
    disclosure of all ingredients; if the ingredients turn out
    to be natural and safe, this is a manufacturer worth
    supporting.

Our Legacy of Natural Health

Vitamins taken alone outside of a healthy diet have never been a
panacea for health and healing. If divorced from a holistic approach,
one that treats the body as a complete system with multiple needs,
vitamins often become nothing more than lubricants in a malfunction-
ing machine.

Holistic medicine, known to us today as a "complementary" or
"integrative" approach to healing, has its botanical roots in the ancient
idea that a healthy plant-based diet and lifestyle, combined with herbal
remedy supplementation, could best support a long life distinguished
by good and robust health. Perhaps the greatest practitioner of this
ancient wisdom tradition was Hippocrates, the fifth century B.C. Greek
physician, who has been credited with saying, "Let thy food by thy
medicine and thy medicine be thy food."

Hippocrates and other innovators of the complementary healing
system examined no part of the human condition in isolation from its
other parts. All aspects of a person's mind and body, including environment and lifestyle influences, came under scrutiny when ailments were
diagnosed and treatments offered. This perspective on the necessity
for treating "wholeness" using herbs and diet was also shared by the
ancient medical systems that arose in Egypt, East India, and China.

The drift away from this reliance on natural botanicals and a philosophy of wholeness and living in balance with nature began when a
germ theory of illness and disease was popularized during the mid-
1800s. Louis Pasteur developed a process of heating substances in high
temperatures to destroy bacteria: pasteurization. This innovation helped
to inspire the idea of a "magic bullet" approach to medicine in which
specific drugs or chemical compounds could be designed to attack the
germs believed to cause disease.

Although this practice worked well to eliminate germs, it never addressed the holistic or systemic root causes of illness and disease. Magic bullets became the holy grail of Western medicine.

Our society's reliance on magic bullets assumes that they treat the entire disease, including its underlying causes, when in fact they are most often treating the symptom of the disease, and with potentially severe side effects, as in the case with chemotherapy. Sadly, we then manufacture and prescribe additional pills to counteract the negative side effects of these initial drugs.

Furthermore, magic-bullet theories also disempower by promoting and perpetuating a myth that we can be instantly "fixed" when we become sick or diseased. Many people, therefore, forsake responsibility for making healthy choices and instead rely on medicine to correct many years of abuse.

As we know, drug companies have benefited most directly from the chemical mania that promised us a better life through chemistry. This harnessing of public imagination has placed these corporations in the top three wealthiest among all industries. Pharmaceutical industry leaders were able to capture much of the newly emerging vitamin industry because they were already synthesizing and developing many drug formulations during the same period. Because they were the only suppliers and promoters of synthetic vitamins, their monopoly allowed them to effectively control the new supplement industry.

More than 50 years of experience with all kinds of people and all sorts of illness and disease at the Hippocrates Health Institute has shown us that the persistent treatment of symptoms without an exploration into and eradication of the root cause of any disease or illness rarely, if ever, results in long-term health and well-being. New integrative approaches to health and healing are required if we are to break free of the synthetics belief system.

If you visit a modern hospital in China or India today you will most likely find that modern facilities are right next door to traditional medical facilities. At their major medical facilities and hospitals you can receive surgery in one ward and herbal remedies or diet recommendations in another—all under the same roof. The integrative approach to medicine is still in its infancy in the Western world, but is becoming more popular as people begin to understand the importance of natural, traditional therapies and how self-responsibility is the central cause of all recovery.

Meet the Natural Vitamin Pioneers

The following are some champions of natural vitamins who have supported the concept of real vitamins and real nutritional values and who rejected the use of synthetic vitamins. Many of these pioneers have been forgotten or ignored, though they still made remarkable contributions toward bringing the consumer better-quality foods and supplements.

Dr. Royal Lee, born on April 7, 1885, was an influential American leader in nutritional science who in the 1930s advocated the use of naturally occurring vitamins. He challenged the prevailing domination of synthetic vitamin producers and the purveyors of synthetic nutrients. He created a successful whole-food supplement company that distributed to natural doctors who had the knowledge to explain the benefits to their patients. One of Dr. Lee's many wise statements was "supplements in and of themselves will never replace a health giving diet—it is only a measure to increase nourishment and prevent disorder."

One of his major interests as a student at Marquette University was nutrition. During his senior year he presented a paper to his class on "The Systemic Causes of Dental Caries," which was written at the age of 16. He outlined the relationship of vitamin deficiency to tooth decay and showed the necessity of vitamins in the diet for normal functioning of the endocrine glands. His research into the food sources of naturally occurring vitamins led to the development of a multiple-vitamin concentrate derived from natural vegetable sources such as defatted wheat (germ), carrot (root), dried alfalfa juice, oat flour, rice bran, and other ingredients. In 1929, he founded the Vitamin Products Company.

Dr. Lee grew up on a farm near Edmund in the southwestern part of Wisconsin. At age 12, he had compiled a notebook on biochemistry and nutrition by copying definitions from the school dictionary. He also began collecting books on these subjects and continued his acute interest throughout the years, resulting in one of the largest individual collections in the world. While still in high school, he taught advanced physics to a class of fifteen. Upon graduation he engaged in various businesses before being drafted by the Army to serve in World War I. At the conclusion of the war and his discharge in 1919, he enrolled in Milwaukee's Marquette University, where he graduated from dental college.

In the early 1920s, Western nations faced a new health threat: coronary heart disease. Dr. Lee knew that vitamins and other nutrients were removed from flour and rice by commercial milling. He believed that this correlated to the increase in heart disease. At about this same time the scientific community was able to isolate vitamins and standardize them as drugs. In effect, the food manufacturers altered and removed the health-sustaining components from the grains and then "fortified" the product by adding synthetic, inert vitamins. The result was a far inferior product, yet the public believed they were getting the "real thing," or even more erroneously, an "improved," enriched product.

Dr. Lee often ran advertisements in newspapers exposing this food fraud. As a result, he spent a great deal of time in court battling the Food and Drug Administration. The FDA used its power and unlimited taxpayer resources to brand Dr. Lee a racketeer simply because he promoted whole, natural, unadulterated foods with their vitamins and minerals intact.

You can see from the following comment by Dr. Lee in 1933 that his perspective was far ahead of the time:

> Candy, all-white sugar or its products, and white flour including its products such as macaroni, spaghetti, crackers, etc., should be absolutely barred from the diet of the child. All these are energy-producing foods that contain no building materials for the body. The consequences of their toleration are susceptibility to infections, enlarged tonsils, carious teeth, unruly dispositions, stunted growth, rickets, maldevelopment and very often permanent damage to many organs of the body (especially the endocrine glands) that depend upon the vitamin supply for their normal function and development.

In 1941, Dr. Lee organized the Lee Foundation for Nutritional Research under a state charter as a nonprofit organization. The purpose of the Lee Foundation was to engage in research and to coordinate and communicate nutritional breakthroughs from laboratories around the world. The foundation was the world's largest clearinghouse for nutritional information for doctors, agriculturists, and homemakers. During its existence, the Lee Foundation disseminated millions of pieces of literature and hundreds of thousands of books on health and nutrition. The foundation dissolved after his death in 1967, but his written works are preserved and made available today by The International Foundation for Nutrition and Health.

Dr. Lee took time in 1947 to coauthor a book with William Hanson entitled *Protomorphology, Study of Cell Autoregulation*, a study of biological growth factors and a survey of the problems of aging. He also provided moral and financial support to such organizations as Natural Associates, American Academy of Applied Nutrition, National Health Federation, and Health Publications, always championing freedom of choice in "the natural way."

Dr. Lee fought against ignorance over the difference between natural and synthetic vitamins. Here is another of his illuminating written statements in that regard:

> Yes, there is a battle going on between those who are trying to promote better nutrition, and the food manufacturers who insist on making products 'worse so that they can be sold for less,' thereby eliminating the competition of more honest and self-respecting producers who would prefer to apply in business the Golden Rule. These commercial interests have the United States Government on their side... (*Washington Post*, October 26, 1949).

The former head of the FDA's Nutrition Division, Dr. Elmer M. Nelson, along with other "experts," testified in a court case a decade ago that degenerative disease, infectious disease, and functional disease could not result from any nutritional deficiency. For years he has battled for the manufacturers of devitalized foods, tried to stem the tide of public opinion against the use of white flour, refined sugar, pasteurized milk, and imitation butter by vigorous prosecution of any maker of any dietary supplement designed to abate the consequences of using such devitalized food, basing his arguments on the thesis that there were no such things as deficiency diseases. Truly, as Dr. Wiley so accurately remarked in his book *The History of a Crime Against the Pure Food Law* (University of Michigan Press, 1930), "the makers of unfit foods have taken possession of Food & Drug enforcement, and have reversed the effect of the law, protecting the criminals that adulterate foods, instead of protecting the public health."

Dr. Weston Price was another influential natural vitamin pioneer. In the 1930s Dr. Price studied isolated villages in Switzerland, Gaelic communities in the Outer Hebrides, Eskimos and Indians of North America, Melanesian and Polynesian South Sea Islanders, African tribes, Australian Aborigines, New Zealand Maori, and the Indians of South America. Wherever he went, Dr. Price, then in his 60s, found that stalwart bodies resistant to disease, beautiful straight teeth free from decay, and fine characters were typical of people with natural diets.

Dr. Price found that these indigenous diets provided at least four times the amount of water-soluble vitamins, calcium, and other minerals, and at least 10 times the amount of fat-soluble vitamins, compared with Western diets. In native populations that adopted diets of "civilized" Western peoples, Dr. Price saw signs of physical degeneration. The importance of good nutrition for mothers during pregnancy has long been recognized, but Dr. Price discovered that these indigenous peoples practiced preconception nutritional programs for *both* parents. Many tribes even required a period of premarital nutrition. The births of children were spaced to permit the mother to regain her full health and strength to assure subsequent offspring of physical excellence. Special foods rich in fat-soluble vitamins A and D were often given to pregnant and lactating women and maturing boys and girls.

The discoveries and conclusion of Dr. Price are presented in his classic volume *Nutrition and Physical Degeneration*, published by the Price Pottinger Nutrition Foundation in 1939. The book contains striking photographs of handsome, healthy people and illustrates the physical degeneration that occurs when humans abandon nourishing, traditional diets in favor of modern convenience foods. Dr. Price's photographs illustrated the difference in facial structure between those on native diets and those whose parents had adopted the "civilized" diets of devitalized processed foods. These indigenous peoples with their fine bodies, homogeneous reproduction, emotional stability, and freedom from degenerative ills are in stark contrast to those subsisting on the impoverished foods of current civilization—sugar, white flour, pasteurized milk, and convenience foods with extenders, synthetics, and other additives.

Before the U.S. Food and Drug Administration came into being there was the Bureau of Chemistry. Until 1912, this bureau was headed by Dr. Harvey W. Wiley, a medical doctor concerned with protecting Americans from chemical synthetics and toxic food processing. Dr. Wiley was the first commissioner of the Food and Drug Administration (FDA). In his *The History of a Crime Against the Pure Food Law*, he wrote:

> No food product in our country would have any trace of benzoic acid, sulfurous acid or sulfites or any alum or saccharin, save for medical purposes. No soft drink would contain caffeine or theobromine. No bleached flour would enter interstate commerce. Our foods and drugs would be wholly without any form of adulteration and misbranding. The health of our people would be vastly improved and their lives greatly extended. The manufacturers of our food supply, and especially the millers, would devote their energies to improving the public health and promoting happiness in every home by the production of whole ground, unbolted cereal flours and meals.

Dr. Bernard Jensen, a naturopathic physician based in California, was another pioneer who promoted the use of whole foods and avoidance of synthetic vitamins and nutrients. Few can aspire to accomplish in a lifetime the international impact he and his work have had on millions of lives.

Dr. Jensen was versed in a wide variety of holistic healthcare disciplines including natural nutrition, bowel care, hydrotherapy, fasting, reflexology, iridology, polarity, glandular balancing, homeopathy, herbs, acupuncture, and craniopathy (the science of cranium-head bone structure and health). Dr. Jensen criticized the tobacco industry and the food giants who indirectly supported the persecution of Dr. Royal Lee and used their advertising to promote wrong and harmful information.

Can you believe that the cigarette ads of the 1940s and '50s actually showed medical doctors promoting the digestive benefits of smoking Camels? Back then, Coca-Cola and other refined-sugar foods were advertised with such foolish statements as: "Science has shown how [refined] sugar can help keep your appetite and weight under control." These revelations came from *Empty Harvest*, a book by Dr. Jensen exposing man's disconnection to the earth.

Dr. Kristine Nolfi, MD, healed herself of breast cancer early in the 20th century by means of raw foods and whole-food nutrients. Dr. Nolfi founded Humlegaarden, a residential natural healthcare clinic near Copenhagen, Denmark. In the 1920s she began a lifelong quest to bring the living-food and whole-food supplement message to Europe. She had a spectacular level of health and focus, and in spite of many roadblocks from her peers in the medical community she succeeded in establishing herself and her clinic as the premier natural hospital of the early 20th century. Her use of germinated and raw foods, a diet she called "the living food program," helped thousands of people in Europe achieve renewed health and well-being and sparked the imagination of health-seekers worldwide. Nolfi's scientific mind helped her develop a road map for natural-health practitioners using raw, living foods, pure water, fresh air, and regular exercise.

Dr. Ann Wigmore, MD, founded a health information center in Massachusetts in the early 1950s (it later became Hippocrates Institute), after healing herself from colon cancer with whole foods and whole-food supplements. Her approach centered on enzyme nutrition through wheatgrass and other sprouts, along with unprocessed and unheated foods and supplements. She believed that nutrition from natural sources was critical to the development of a strong immune system and a healthy body, mind, and spirit. Dr. Wigmore was one of the world's most outspoken advocates of unadulterated supplements for the use of achieving lifelong health.

The renowned Danish healer Alma Nissen was afflicted by crippling arthritis at an early age. She healed it completely with a natural diet and lifestyle, and, after studying natural medicine, founded the Brandal Health Clinic near Stockholm, Sweden. People from all over the world attended her clinic, which treated all forms of illness: arthritis, asthma, cardiovascular diseases, dermal maladies such as eczema and psoriasis, and autoimmune disorders. Her general protocol was organic whole foods and whole-food supplements. The Swedish government conducted extensive studies on patient results via Linköping University Hospital in Linköping, Sweden, and found that there was a more-than-90-percent reduction in, and reversal of, the aforementioned disorders when the participants adhered to the strict nutrition-based program. Alma Nissen, a pioneer in the field of nutritional science, was respected by Scandinavia's medical community.

Today many health professionals, nutritional instructors, and advocates encourage the use of truly natural vitamin supplementation from pure food sources. These men and women are upholding the hallowed tradition of pure, natural food nutrition that has been pioneered for the benefit of humanity.

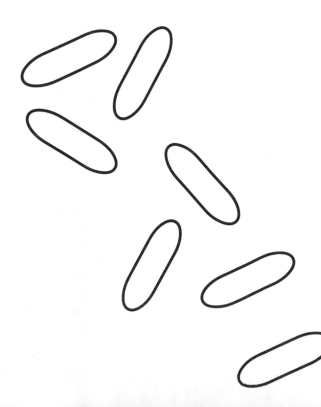

— PART II —

WHAT SUPPLEMENTS REALLY DO FOR YOU

CHAPTER 5

FATTY ACIDS AND FISH FALLACIES

Fatty Acids

Food supplementation fads come and go like the seasons as various industries manipulate the popular imagination by touting their products as the latest solution to whatever health ailment has been identified as the newest "epidemic" to afflict us.

Fish oil supplements containing omega-3 fatty acids illustrate one of the more recent campaigns to win the hearts, minds, and paychecks of consumers. The omega-3 fatty acids cannot be produced by the human body but are necessary for our mental and physical functioning. They have gradually been replaced in the average human diet by omega-6 fatty acids from unhealthy sources such as meat, corn oil, and other cooking oils.

One result of our omega-3 deficiency has been an upsurge in the incidence of depression. Though we can get our omega-3s from healthy sources such as walnuts and dark leafy vegetables, if we consume enough of them, manufacturers of fish oil supplements have promoted their products as the primary antidote to the omega-3 shortage in our foods.

Many health concerns and problems are associated with this fish oil campaign and need to be exposed. But first, here is a little more background on the role omega-3 plays in our lives.

The research on essential fatty acids (EFAs) like omega-3s continues to attest to their complexity and essential role in human health and development. Not only are they shown to support immune function, cardiovascular health, vision, memory, and mood stabilization, but they are also essential for optimum fetal growth.

Two categories of essential fatty acids, omega-6 and omega-3, are not made in the body and must be obtained through the diet for health. These fatty acids are necessary to maintain cell membranes, transport fats in the body, and aid in the production of prostaglandins.

Omega-3 fatty acids are needed for the health of our brain, nerves, skin, and circulatory and immune functions. Studies have shown that omega-3s are helpful in preventing or treating health conditions such as arthritis, cancer, heart disease, multiple sclerosis, fibromyalgia, weight gain, ADD/ADHD, Alzheimer's, allergies, depression, strokes, diabetes, skin problems, and many other concerns.

Clinical evidence indicates that omega-3 can help improve our health and prevent diseases. For example, omega-3 may be useful in the prevention and treatment of Alzheimer's by preventing Alzheimer's brain lesions. The USDA has updated the Food Guide Pyramid to include omega-3 in the "healthy fats" section, while revising outdated and inaccurate charts that promote large quantities of meat and dairy products. Guidelines from the various heart associations have also been revised to include omega-3 oils.

Unlike the saturated fats found in animal products like lard and butter, omega-3 fatty acids are polyunsaturated. *Saturated* and *polyunsaturated* refers to the number of hydrogen atoms attached to the carbon chain of the fatty acid. Polyunsaturated fats, unlike saturated fats, are liquid at room temperature and remain liquid when refrigerated or frozen. Monounsaturated fats, found in olive oil for example, are liquid at room temperature but harden when refrigerated. When eaten in appropriate amounts, each type of fat can contribute to health. However, the importance of omega-3 fatty acids to both health promotion and disease prevention is unique.

The three most nutritionally important omega-3 fatty acids are alpha-linolenic acid, eicosapentaenoic acid (EPA), and docosahexaenoic acid (DHA). Alpha-linolenic acid is one of two fatty acids classified as essential. The other essential fatty acid is an omega-6 fatty acid called linoleic acid. Both are classified as essential because the human body is unable to manufacture them on its own and because they play a fundamental role in vital physiological functions. Therefore, we must be sure our diet contains sufficient amounts of omegas.

There are plenty of dietary sources of omega-3 fatty acids to choose from. One of the most popular sources is now animal flesh, which we do not recommend at all. Here is why. For starters, there are many good vegetable sources of omega-3s: chia seed, raspberry seeds, pumpkin seeds, walnuts, hemp seeds, flax seeds, sprouts, algae, and dark green leafy vegetables such as kale.

Essential fatty acids such as those found in omega-3s are the "good fats" you hear about these days. Good fats compete with bad fats, so it is important to eliminate transfats and hydrogenated fats, like margarine or high-cholesterol fats (animal fat), while consuming enough good fats. Good fats raise your HDL, or "good cholesterol." One of the jobs of this high-density lipoprotein (HDL), or good cholesterol, is to grab your "bad cholesterol," LDL (low density lipoprotein), and escort it to the liver where it is broken down and eliminated.

Essential fatty acids (EFAs) like omega-3s are necessary fats that humans cannot synthesize, so they must be obtained through our diet. EFAs support the cardiovascular, reproductive, immune, and nervous systems. The human body also needs EFAs to manufacture and repair cell membranes, enabling the cells to obtain optimum nutrition and expel harmful waste products.

A primary function of EFAs like omega-3s is to regulate body functions such as heart rate, blood pressure, blood clotting, fertility, and conception. They help immune function by regulating inflammation and encouraging the body to fight infections. EFAs like omega-3s are also needed for proper growth in children, particularly for neural development and maturation of sensory systems. Fetuses and breast-fed infants also require an adequate supply of EFAs derived from a healthy mother.

Omega-3 deficiency or imbalance is linked with serious health conditions—heart attacks, cancer, insulin resistance, asthma, lupus, schizophrenia, depression, postpartum depression, accelerated aging, stroke, obesity, diabetes, arthritis, ADD/ADHD, and Alzheimer's disease, among others.

It is thought by many health professionals, such as Dr. Daniel Amen, an assistant clinical professor of psychiatry and human behavior at the University of California, Irvine School of Medicine, that the epidemic attention deficit disorder (ADD) is in large part due to omega-3 (DHA) deficiency in children. Dr. Amen's groundbreaking work into these maladies has revolutionized the field's understanding on treatment. It is absolutely crucial for fetuses and infants to ingest it for proper brain and nerve development. Arthritis pain and even cancer can result from the repeated unchecked circulation of stress-related toxic biochemicals as well as from free radicals and other toxins. Omega-3s help reduce the buildup of these toxins, thereby reducing the risk of serious diseases.

Omega-3s are found in green and blue algae, chia seed, flaxseed oil and meal, raspberry seeds, primrose oil, hempseed oil, hempseeds, walnuts, pumpkin seeds, Brazil nuts, sesame seeds, avocados, dark leafy green vegetables like kale, spinach, mustard and collard greens, and a wide variety of germinated seeds, nuts, and grains.

The Fish Fallacy

Omega-3s are also found in other sources that we do not recommend, such as canola oil, fish oils, salmon, mackerel, sardines, anchovies, albacore tuna and other fish, and such marine animals as seals and dolphins. We hear much talk about the benefits of eating oily fish, especially because many oily fish contain significant amounts of omega-3s. But are fish oils really good and safe for you?

Remember the stories about mothers giving their children daily doses of cod liver oil as a food supplement for health? Maybe 70 years ago, our oceans, lakes, and streams were clean-water resources where you could find clean fish, but today they are pools of toxins. Our air and soil are as horribly polluted as our water resources and the creatures that inhabit them.

Commercial tuna is one of the most polluted fish you could possibly eat. The U.S. and other governments are recommending a deep reduction in tuna consumption because all tuna tested so far contains unsafe amounts of mercury and other heavy metals. Mercury toxicity affects the human central nervous system functioning, including brain function and nerve atrophy, which causes many related diseases.

According to a report by Finnish researchers, middle-aged men should avoid eating fish high in mercury (such as salmon, flounder, mackerel, cod, lobster, and shrimp) because it could put them at a greater risk for heart attacks and other heart ailments. Researchers from the University of Kuopio in Finland monitored the health and diet of 2,682 Finnish men between the ages of 42 and 60 and found that they had a 50- to 70-percent higher risk of having a heart attack, heart disease, or cardiovascular disease if they had elevated levels of mercury. Another study published in the *American Heart Association Journal* found that men with high levels of mercury increase their risk of heart disease by 60 percent and the risk of dying of a heart attack by 70 percent. ("Middle-aged men should avoid eating fish high in mercury because it could put them at greater risk for heart attacks and other heart ailments," by Joan Lowy, Scripps Howard News Service, February 1, 2005.)

The story of tuna is the same for salmon, cod, and other fish used to produce fish oils containing omega-3s. Farm-grown fish now contain even higher levels of heavy metals than those in the wild. This occurs in part because farmers feed the captive fish ground-up fishmeal from other highly toxic fish. Farmers must also administer large doses of antibiotics to combat rampant disease and high rates of mortality due to viruses and bacteria. Disease is excessive in these pools; they are unnaturally crowded and highly overpopulated, lacking sufficient oxygen to keep microbes at normal levels. Additionally, practices to enhance the marketability of certain fish are alarmingly unnatural. Farm-raised salmon, severely lacking the nourishment provided by their natural habitats, are being injected with dyes to change their otherwise white flesh to the pink shade consumers expect. Factory farming has been created to meet the demand for foods, and it has had significant and often unhealthy effects not only on the food itself but also on our environment.

We also find many fish contaminated with ciguatera poisoning, which has been implicated in chronic fatigue syndrome. The ciguatera toxin originates in the algae eaten by small reef fish, which are then eaten by larger fish that are then consumed by humans.

We never recommend fish-oil supplementation or any fish flesh. As we have also said, farmed-raised fish are highly polluted with dyes, poor quality, and even contaminated feeds, run-off from soil contamination that pollutes our waters, and an internal biochemical contamination caused by the stress of crowding.

Why Fish Oils Are Hazardous to Your Health

Lipid peroxide contamination is a condition in which fish oils have oxidized (the oil molecules are destroyed through the exposure to oxygen) and become rancid, cancer-causing fats. This poisoning occurs to some degree when fish oils are exposed to air for any period of time, and further complicates the alleged health benefits of fish oil consumption.

When rancid fishmeal and rancid fats are fed in large quantities to fish on fish farms, fat degeneration develops, yet another reason why rancid "farmed" fish-oil is carcinogenic.

The only reason that fish oil is known as an "accepted" source of omega-3 fats is because of the extensive marketing and lobbying investments made by the fish industry. Throughout the years the public, and professionals who do not take the time to study the basic science, have been led to believe that fish and their byproducts are good food sources. This began in the 1990s when red meat received bad press after being linked to heart disease and high cholesterol and high blood pressure. The fish industry capitalized on the negative press by trumpeting the message that consuming fish and other fish products was a healthy alternative to red meat. This is a dangerous myth.

Two hormone precursors that stimulate the production of cortisone in the body are EPA and DHA, which come naturally from plant-based foods. This is an essential body function: The body is designed to produce essential nutrients like EPA and DHA from whole foods and naturally occurring supplements. When you take EPA and DHA from fish oil sources you are bypassing a natural metabolic pathway in your body, with potentially grave long-term effects. One negative side effect is the atrophy of our body's natural EPA and DHA production systems. It is not only harmful, but it also makes no sense to purchase and consume a substance that is naturally produced by one's own body. The only groups that profit are the makers of these toxic fish-oil substances.

About 50 years ago, it was found that a large amount of cod liver oil in dogs' diets increased their death rate from cancer by 20 times. Also, a diet rich in fish oil causes intense production of toxic lipid peroxides, and has been observed to reduce a man's sperm count to zero.

Another problem with fish oils is rancidity. When a fish dies out of the water—in an oxygenated environment—its oils become almost immediately rancid and unusable for omega-3 purposes. The problem is that fish oil is very unstable, and begins to oxidize or decay as soon as it is extracted from the fish and exposed to oxygen, light, or heat. These rancid oils are known carcinogens.

Many fish-oil processors mask the dead-fish smell of the rancid oils by filtering them and adding preservatives and antioxidants such as synthesized vitamin E and ascorbic acid (synthetic vitamin C). Then they seal the fish oils in capsules so you cannot smell them. I have opened capsules of fish oils and the odor is always there—a sure sign of rancid oil. When fish oil is filtered, preserved, and "deodorized," it is very carcinogenic. High doses of fish oils can actually cause your body to emit a slightly fishy odor. There are many superior vegetable sources high in omega-3s from plants that have their own naturally occurring antioxidant matrix.

Fish and fish oils contain mercury. Data from the Center for Disease Control indicates that nearly 10 percent of women of childbearing age in the United States have unsafe mercury levels. This number is higher in countries where more fish is eaten. The major contributor to the body's mercury burden, according to multiple studies, is the mercury found in fish and fish oils. High mercury levels have been linked to infertility, high blood pressure, and neurological, endocrine, and other concerns.

It is also important to know as a consumer that fish oils are often used in margarine and other shortenings you may be consuming. They are widely used as a lubricant in soap-making and in paint. Sometimes "fish oil" is mislabeled on a product, and the oil may actually come from seals or marine mammals such as dolphins. Seal oil is very high in omega-3s, but do you want to eat dolphins or seals?

Tests by a team of New Zealand researchers found that many fish-oil samples contain oxidative byproducts, indicating the oil is degrading even further and becoming increasingly rancid within the capsule. Fish oils are often processed by mincing the whole fish and then extracting the oil with chemical solvents and heat. Heat processing and solvent residues will only serve to create more carcinogenic substances. Eating fish oil is dangerous and promotes disease rather than prevents it.

Think about it. You would not eat spoiled and rancid fish. So why would you eat spoiled and rancid fish oil, which happens every time you consume fish-oil capsules?

Fish oils contain the long chain n-3 derivatives EPA and DHA. These n-3 derivatives are up to 25 times more sensitive to destruction by light, oxygen, and heat than health-promoting vegetable oils. Fish oils are more likely to contain an even higher percentage of damaged molecules than one would find in fine vegetable oils.

Most people fail to consider that fish oils are prone to the same pollution as the fish flesh they come from. Not only is damage done to the fish oil during processing, but there are concerns about fish oil contamination by pesticides, mercury, dioxins, and chlorinated pesticides. The removal of these toxins requires more processing, with accumulated destruction to the fish oil molecules along the way. Better to use only fresh vegetable sources of omega-3s.

Flaxseed oil has been prescribed for health benefits long before anyone conjured up the myth of fish oil as a good source for omega-3s. Flax oil has been used to promote health as far back as 650 B.C., when Hippocrates, the father of Western medicine, advised eating flax to help relieve inflamed mucous membranes and to ameliorate abdominal conditions.

A word about the recent fad of consuming unhealthy canola oil for omega-3s: Canola oil (rapeseed oil) is poisonous to many living things: it is an excellent insect repellent. We have been using it, in a highly diluted form, to kill the aphids on our plants. It works well for this, but not as a food. In fact, canola oil was once used only for machinery lubrication, as a fuel, for soap and synthetic rubber productions, and as an illuminate for color pages in magazines. It definitely has its place as industrial oil, but it has no value on your kitchen shelf as a food, or, for that matter, in foods on the shelves in our grocery stores.

Canola oil started being used as a food when someone discovered that it was cheap to grow and process and did not have saturated fat content. For those reasons, it soon became very popular. Today, many baked goods on grocery shelves contain canola oil. Motor oil contains no saturated fats either, but does that mean you will start putting motor oil on your salad? As a non-food, canola oil is not a suitable source of omega-3s.

Some possible side effects of canola-oil consumption may include loss of vision, disruption of the central nervous system, respiratory illness, anemia, constipation, increased incidence of heart disease and cancer, low birth weights in infants, and irritability.

Vegetable Sources of Omega-3s

The vegetable sources of omega-3s we've listed also contain naturally occurring antioxidants, such as vitamin C, vegetable vitamin E, tannins, and other related antioxidants that help to prevent rancidity.

Adding preservatives and antioxidants to fish oil to help prevent the rancidity of any remaining omega-3s and other nutrients does not help. Even when fish-oil omega-3 parts are preserved, unpreserved rancid parts that are dangerously carcinogenic are still left behind.

This is not true when preserving omega-3s containing vegetable oils, such as raspberry seed oil or pumpkin seed oil. These vegetable sources of omega-3 do not have to be preserved with vitamin E or other antioxidants to prevent them from becoming rancid. They already contain naturally occurring vitamin E and other antioxidants that ensure preservation for long periods when stored in airtight containers.

Given the contamination issues with fish and fish oils, the rancidity of fish oil, and documented immune-system suppression, only uneducated or misinformed individuals would call fish or fish oils health food! The safest and healthiest option is to avoid fish oils entirely and use only vegetable-based products for your omega-3 nutritional requirements.

CHAPTER 6

THE HEALTH ROLES OF SPECIFIC VITAMINS

Your Body's Four Vitamin Musketeers

"All for one and one for all" might well be a theme for your body's four Vitamin Musketeers—A, D, E, and K—because these nutrients are intertwined with our consumption of natural food sources, and all work together to keep our physical defenses strong against illness and disease. All four can provide us with their benefits only if we consume a range of mostly dark green vegetables and freshwater algae, though vitamin D does also come to us free of charge from sunshine.

Attempts to synthesize these vitamins in laboratories to extract the "magic bullet" active ingredient have mostly produced variations on Frankenstein's monster. By eliminating all of the nutrient cofactors from natural foods that support the functions of these vitamins, synthetics present us with mere shadows of the real thing, more like a drug than one of nature's crowning achievements.

To evaluate the differences between natural and synthetic versions of the four Vitamin Musketeers, start with vitamin A, which is necessary for a range of bodily functions such as normal cell division and growth, embryonic development, DNA synthesis, and for maintaining the mucous membranes of the respiratory, digestive, and urinary tracts. It is also vital for good eyesight because it plays a key role in converting light into electrical signals, and protects against damage caused by free radicals. A deficiency of vitamin A causes a generalized drying up of mucous membranes and greatly increases the risk of infection, as well as resulting in an inability to see in low light—a condition known as night blindness.

Beta-carotene is a vitamin A precursor, which the body uses to create complete vitamin A. Carrots, sunflower sprouts, red peppers, mangos, cantaloupes, cabbage, broccoli sprouts, as well as green leafy vegetables such as spinach and kale, are foods that are rich in this nutrient. Usually, the more intense the color of the fruit or vegetable, the more beta carotene it contains. Naturally occurring beta carotene, not retinol, is the real vitamin A precursor along with its associated carotenoid factors that the body can convert into a usable form of vitamin A. Naturally occurring vitamin A and beta carotene are well-documented immune boosters and cancer fighters. They are also known for their role as antioxidants.

Synthetic vitamin A, by contrast, may actually bring about *in-creases* in certain types of cancer. *The New England Journal of Medicine* reported on April 14, 1994 ("The Effect of Vitamin E and Beta Carotene on the Incidence of Lung Cancer and Other Cancer in Male Smokers") the results of a 10-year large-scale study in Finland. This was a randomized and double-blind trial to determine whether daily supplementation of (synthetic) vitamin E and (synthetic) beta-carotene (vitamin A) would reduce the incidence of lung and other cancers. The study included 29,133 male smokers 50 to 69 years of age. Major newspapers headlined the findings as evidence that supplements aren't effective in preventing cancer.

This study showed conclusively that synthetic vitamin A (synthetic beta-carotene) had no antioxidant effect whatsoever. A true antioxidant, such as vitamin A from a food source, helps to protect heart muscle, lungs, and artery surfaces from breaking down prematurely. In this study, the subjects who received the synthetic beta-carotene actually had an 8-percent-higher incidence of fatal heart attacks, strokes, and lung cancer than those who used the placebo. The synthetic vitamin A brought no vitamin activity to the tissues that needed it.

Pharmacologic doses (high amounts of isolated chemicals) of synthetic beta-carotenes (chemically made, not naturally occurring carotenes from foods such as carrots or green vegetables) were found to block the antioxidant activity of the other 50 naturally occurring carotenoids in a nutritious diet at a dosage of only 20 mgs per day. Anti-cancer activity, therefore, was stopped in its tracks by the synthetic carotene supplements. As a toxic chemical introduced into the body, the synthetic vitamin A further stressed the immune system, the liver, and the kidneys; all were forced to work harder to break down this chemical compound in order to remove it from the body.

Synthetic Vitamin A and Toxicity

Vitamin A was discovered in 1919, and by 1924 it had been broken down and separated from its natural whole-food complex and "purified." By 1931, a major pharmaceutical company had succeeded in "synthesizing" vitamin A—meaning that the company had created a purely chemical copy of a fraction of naturally occurring vitamin A. Naturally occurring vitamin A works with an entire group of other components, such as:

- Retinols.
- Retinoids.
- Retinal.
- Carotenoids.
- Carotenes.
- Fatty acids.
- Vitamin C.
- Vitamin E.
- Vitamin B.
- Vitamin D.
- Enzymes.
- Minerals.
- Hormones.
- Oxygen.

Isolated from these other factors, synthetic vitamin A is a fraction of the real thing that cannot perform its biological functions. Taken as a synthetic supplement, it must draw on this list of nutrients already in the body in order to complete its makeup. The naturally occurring vitamin A matrix is already complete and ready to activate its function.

Some synthetic vitamin A consists only of retinol or retinoic acid. The well-publicized potential for toxicity with mega doses of vitamin A often involves one of these three. Vitamin A toxicity, known as hypervitaminosis, always results from an excess of synthetic, "purified" vitamin A, and never from a naturally occurring food source of vitamin A.

So although synthetic vitamins mimic benefits in some instances, they have an overall negative net effect on your health.

Effects of vitamin A toxicity include:

◌ Tumor enhancement.

◌ Joint disorders.

◌ Osteoporosis.

◌ Extreme dryness of eyes, mouth, and skin.

◌ Enlargement of liver and spleen.

◌ Immune suppression.

◌ Birth defects.

Vitamin A is found naturally in hemp oil, all green sprouts, avocado, blue-green algae and green algae, and sea vegetables. Vegetable sources of the vitamin A precursor called beta-carotene are the best choice. Beta-carotene comes from carrots, pumpkins, sweet potatoes, winter squashes, cantaloupes, pink grapefruit, apricots, and spinach. As we have said, the more intense the color of a fruit or vegetable, the higher its beta-carotene content.

Results of two national surveys, the third *National Health and Nutrition Examination Survey* (NHANES III 1988–91) and the *Continuing Survey of Food Intakes by Individuals* (CSFII 1994), produced evidence that dietary intake often does not meet recommended levels for vitamin A. Interestingly, there is no current Recommended Daily Allowance for beta-carotene or other vitamin A carotenoids.

Vitamin D (3) (Cholecalciferol)

In 1922, Edward Mellanby discovered vitamin D while research-ing the bone disease rickets. Nicknamed the "sunshine vitamin" be-cause it can be produced by the exposure of the skin to the sun, as well as to full-spectrum ultraviolet rays, vitamin D is needed by our bodies to absorb calcium and phosphorus. It is also vital to healthy bones and teeth. Our research at Hippocrates has revealed that a shocking 40 percent of the general population is lacking in adequate levels of vita-min D. However, there is only a small margin between safe and toxic levels of this vitamin, and excess can cause kidney damage.

Vitamin D is currently known as a pro-hormone involved in min-eral metabolism and bone growth. Its most dramatic effect is to facili-tate intestinal absorption of calcium, although it also stimulates absorption of phosphate and magnesium. In the absence of vitamin D, dietary calcium is not absorbed efficiently. Vitamin D stimulates the expression of a number of proteins involved in transporting calcium from the lumen of the intestine across the epithelial cells and into blood.

The term *vitamin D* (synthetic) actually refers to a group of steroid molecules. Naturally occurring vitamin D3, also known as cholecalcif-erol, is generated in the skin of humans and animals when light energy is absorbed by a precursor molecule 7-dehydrocholesterol. Those with adequate exposure to sunlight, who are generally healthy, do not nor-mally require dietary supplementation of vitamin D.

Vitamin D is called the "sunshine vitamin" because the body will produce sufficient vitamin D when the skin is exposed to the sun two or three times weekly for as little as 15 minutes. Vitamin D is essential for the absorption and use of calcium in our bodies and for mainte-nance of strong bones; it is also now known as the most important nutrient in preventing osteoporosis and in reversing depression. Vita-min D is a fat-soluble vitamin that is stored in the body fat and re-leased as required.

The yeast form of vitamin D, called vitamin D2 or ergosterol, is made by artificially irradiating fungus in an exposure process. Vitamin D from ergosterol is not a naturally occurring form of vitamin D. It is manmade for consumption as a vitamin D supplement. Ergosterol is often used as the vitamin D source in fortified foods and food supplements.

Biologists knew as far back as 1936 that synthesized ergosterol forms of vitamin D were inferior to naturally occurring forms of vitamin D: "A recent report states that the whole-food unit of natural vitamin D is about 100 times more potent in protecting chickens and children from rickets than the incomplete unit of irradiated ergosterol," read one such reference from a May 1936 article titled "The Influence of Milk Constituents on the Effectiveness of Vitamin D" by G. Supplee, S. Ansbacher, R. Bender, and G. Flanigan, in the journal *Biological Chemistry.*

By 1937, scientists also knew that synthetic vitamin D might put women's offspring at risk for birth defects. Reported the *Ohio State Medical Journal*:

> Among 90 women who received viosterol (a synthesized form of vitamin D) and calcium lactate, the placenta showed calcification 'beyond normal expectation or experience'.... Fetal heads were less moulded, suture lines less distinct and general appearance of ossification or post-maturity was noted. Labors were prolonged... (W. Brehm, "Potential dangers of viosterol during pregnancy with observations of calcification of placentae").

Naturally occurring vitamin D in foods is scarce. Fresh-water algae, sea vegetables, shitake mushrooms, and edible weeds are the vegetable sources highest in naturally occurring vitamin D. In years past it was common, although undesirable and unhealthy, for mothers to give their children cod liver oil daily to avert a concern over rickets. Vitamin D deficiency was such a problem among many children that governments mandated that all milk be fortified with synthetic vitamin D. Unfortunately to this day most milk and other dairy products are still fortified with vitamin D. Although milk and its related products should never be consumed, the majority of the population still believes it to be a necessary food. (For support of this statement, read Cornell University biochemist T. Colin Campbell's book, *The China Study*, BenBella Books, 2006.) The best naturally occurring source of vitamin D is still made by the body in response to sunshine and full-spectrum lighting.

Adequate vitamin D is necessary for health, but consuming large quantities of synthetic vitamin D is dangerous. A single dose of synthetic vitamin D of 50 mg or greater is toxic for adults. The immediate effect of an overdose of vitamin D is abdominal cramps, nausea, and vomiting. Toxic doses of vitamin D taken with time may result in a buildup of irreversible deposits of calcium crystals in the soft tissues of the body that damage the heart, lungs, and kidneys.

Vitamin E

In 1922, University of California researchers Herbert Evans and Katherine Bishop discovered vitamin E in green leafy vegetables. Experiments in that year showed that rats reared exclusively on whole milk grew normally but were sterile and could not reproduce. Evans and Bishop showed that the missing factor was vitamin E, an antioxidant, which is abundant in certain foods such as green leaves and wheat grass. Natural forms of vitamin E (complex) lose up to 99 percent of their potency when separated from their natural synergists (naturally occurring matrix factors).

Synthetic vitamin E is *not* true vitamin E.

Vitamin E is fat-soluble and exists in eight different naturally occurring forms: four tocopherols (including alpha, beta, gamma, and delta), and four tocotrienols (also alpha, beta, gamma, and delta). Each form has its own biological activity. Alpha-tocopherol is the main recognized form of vitamin E, the form found in the largest quantities in the blood and tissue. Because alpha-tocopherol appears to have a significant nutritional activity, it is the part of the vitamin that most people identify as vitamin E.

Alpha-tocopherol is a powerful biological antioxidant and acts to protect our cells against the effects of free radicals, those damaging byproducts of the body's metabolism. Free radicals cause cell damage that very often contributes to the development of cardiovascular disease, cancer, and premature aging.

In the case of vitamin E (tocopherol), the dextro form occurs in nuts, seeds, grains, legumes, and vegetables, and is the form that is highly usable and biologically active in the body. Synthetic vitamin E, found in the levo-form of tocopherol (listed as dl-tocopherol), is often made from a petrochemical and is not usable by the body, so our systems must work to eliminate it. This is a synthetic fraction divided from its other parts, so it is not authentic vitamin E. As is the case with all natural vitamins, vitamin E is a complex of naturally occurring tocopherols and other naturally occurring factors and cofactors that cannot work effectively in isolation.

Fats, which are an integral part of all cell membranes, are vulnerable to destruction through oxidation by free radicals. The fat-soluble vitamin alpha-tocopherol helps to intercept free radicals, preventing a chain reaction of lipid (fat) destruction. Aside from maintaining the integrity of cell membranes throughout the body, alpha-tocopherol is known to protect dense fats in low-density lipoproteins (LDLs) from oxidation. Lipoproteins are particles composed of lipids and proteins, which are able to transport fats through the blood stream untouched. LDL transports healthy cholesterol from the liver to the tissues of the body. Oxidized LDLs have been implicated in the development of cardiovascular diseases. Alpha-tocopherol is known to inhibit the activity of the protein kinase C, an important cell-signaling molecule, as well as to affect the expression and activity of immune and inflammatory cells.

Vitamin E deficiency has been associated with severe malnutrition, genetic defects affecting the a-tocopherol transfer protein, and fat absorption problems. Children with cystic fibrosis or cholestatic liver disease, who have an impaired capacity to absorb dietary fat and therefore fat-soluble vitamins, may develop symptomatic vitamin E deficiency. Severe vitamin E deficiency results mainly in neurological symptoms such as impaired balance and coordination, and muscle weakness. The developing nervous system appears to be especially vulnerable to vitamin E deficiency, because children born with severe vitamin E deficiency and not treated with whole-food vitamin E may rapidly develop neurological symptoms. In contrast, individuals who develop malabsorption of vitamin E in adulthood may not develop neurological symptoms for 10 to 20 years.

Researchers have noted that oxidative modification of LDL cholesterol (often referred to as "bad" cholesterol) promotes blockages in coronary arteries, which may lead to atherosclerosis and heart attacks. Vitamin E may help prevent or delay coronary heart disease by limiting the oxidation of LDL cholesterol. Vitamin E also may help prevent the formation of blood clots, which lead to heart attack and stroke.

Observational studies have associated lower rates of heart disease with higher vitamin E intake. A study of approximately 90,000 nurses suggested that the incidence of heart disease was 30 to 40 percent lower among nurses with the highest intake of vitamin E from diet. The range of intakes from both diet and natural supplements in this group was 21.6 to 1,000 IU (32 to 1,500 mg), with the median intake being 208 IU (139 mg).

Synthetic alpha-tocopherol is different from natural alpha-tocopherol. Synthetic, chemically created alpha-tocopherol is a combination of eight different isomers, whereas natural alpha-tocopherol is only found as one isomer (RRR-alpha-tocopherol or d-alpha-tocopherol). Actually, only 12.5 percent of synthetic vitamin E is RRR or d-alpha-tocopherol. The body absorbs the natural alpha-tocopherol (RRR or d) the best. Because the synthetic form includes eight isomers (also called allrac or dl-alpha-tocopherol), the body cannot absorb and utilize the other isomers as readily as the RRR-alpha-tocopherol. This results in a decreased bioavilability of synthetic versus natural.

Research conducted at the National Research Council of Canada, a government-sponsored organization, has shown that in humans the natural form is actually two times as bioavailable (digestible) as the synthetic form (reported in Burton G.W., M.G. Traber, R.V. Acuff, et al., "Human plasma and tissue a-tocopherol concentrations in response to supplementation with deuterated natural and synthetic vitamin E," *American Journal of Clinical Nutrition* 67:669–684 [1998]; and Acuff, R.V., R.G. Dunsworth, L.W. Webb, et al., "Transport of dueterium-labeled tocopherols during pregnancy," *American Journal of Clinical Nutrition* 67:459–464 [1998]).

Vitamin E is found naturally in wheat grass, corn, nuts, seeds, olives, spinach, asparagus, green leafy vegetables, uncooked vegetable oils, and every green sprout.

Vitamin K

Not all vitamins were discovered as a cure for a deficiency. Vitamin K's existence was suspected in 1929, but it was discovered, identified, and isolated later, and has been used widely since 1939. Vitamin K was initially unveiled in experiments on chickens. It was found that with certain diets chickens lost their blood-clotting ability. It was observed that the blood of chickens coagulated faster on diets that contained sprouted soybeans containing naturally occurring vitamin K. We now understand that vitamin K has excellent blood-clotting ability. Healthy bacteria in the intestines normally produce vitamin K. Much of the population lacks healthy levels of intestinal "flora" and would be advised to supplement vitamin K through naturally occurring sources. Vitamin K is most readily found in leafy vegetables such as spinach and kale, and to a lesser extent in sprouts and algae, olive oil, and green tea. (We only recommend decaffeinated green tea at Hippocrates.)

Vitamin K is essential for synthesizing the liver protein that controls clotting. It is involved in creating prothrombin, the precursor to thrombin, an important factor for blood clotting, assisting in the production of six of the 13 known proteins needed for clotting. People taking anticoagulants must be careful to keep their vitamin K intake stable. This vitamin is also important to bone formation.

Consuming low levels of vitamin K has been linked with poor bone density, while supplementation with vitamin K has shown improvements in biochemical measures of bone health. A report from the Nurses' Health Study published by the *American Journal of Clinical Nutrition* (Volume 69:74–79) in 1999 suggests that women who get at least 110 micrograms of vitamin K a day are 30 percent less likely to break a hip as women who receive any amount less than 110 micrograms.

Another report from the Nurses' Health Study published by the *American Journal of Clinical Nutrition* (71:1201–1208) in 2000 showed that those eating a daily serving of lettuce or other green leafy vegetable cut the risk of hip fracture in half when compared with eating one serving a week. Data from the Framingham Heart Study also shows an association between high vitamin K intake and reduced risk of hip fracture.

Dietary fat is necessary for the absorption of vitamin K. According to a survey in 1996, a substantial number of people, particularly children and young adults, are not getting the vitamin K they require. A deficiency of vitamin K may result in internal hemorrhaging or nosebleeds. In newborn children a deficiency of vitamin K can result in hemorrhagic disease, as well as postoperative bleeding. As a result, mothers who are breastfeeding need to consume foods that are rich in vitamin K so that the infant is properly nourished.

Toxicity does not easily occur with a normal dietary intake of naturally occurring vitamin K, but synthetic vitamin K can cause a serious toxic reaction. High uptake of synthetic vitamin K in the range of 10,000 mgs or more has been seen to cause flushing and sweating, jaundice, and anemia. Vitamin K-3 (menadione) supplements have been banned by the FDA because of their high toxicity. If you are taking any anti-coagulant (to prevent blood clotting) medication you must consult your medical practitioner before taking a vitamin K–rich supplement of any kind.

Dietary deficiency is rare, but can occur when the body does not absorb fat properly, as in gall-bladder disease. Major sources of vitamin K include spinach, lettuce, broccoli, cauliflower and cabbage, sprouts (specifically onion sprouts), and raw sauerkraut. As a dietary supplement, we recommend a full-spectrum botanical source of vitamin K such as spinach or kale extract.

Your Body's B-Vitamin Extended Family

Your body's family of B vitamins was originally thought of as a single vitamin because the nutritional roles that each plays are very similar. B vitamins are water-soluble (with the exception of B12 stemming from soil-based bacteria), and the body lacks the ability to store them. Any surplus is excreted in the urine.

The B-complex vitamins are a group of eight "officially recognized" vitamins, four other unofficially recognized nutrients, and many still-unknown factors. The eight known vitamin B Complex parts are thiamine (B1), riboflavin (B2), niacin (B3), pantothenic acid (B5), pyridoxine (B6), biotin (B7), folic acid (B9), and cobalamin (B12). All of these provide the body with essential nutrients that are critical to our health.

Each of the B numbers is based on the order in which the specific vitamin part was discovered. This complex only works completely as a real, whole B vitamin family when accompanied by naturally occurring associated factors. Most people cannot obtain enough B vitamins from their daily food sources because today's highly processed foods are virtually devoid of them. Many doctors and nutritionists therefore suggest taking the B-complex vitamins as a supplement group for overall good health and the prevention of nutrient deficiencies.

B-complex vitamins are necessary for:

1. Cell reproduction. Whenever your body needs new cells for the normal functions of metabolism, and for replacements from injury and sickness, vitamin B helps your body reproduce the needed cells and tissue.

2. Nervous system health. Deficiency may cause memory loss and lower reaction time.

3. Heart health. A study conducted among more than 80,000 female nurses was the first to show a direct link between these B vitamins, folate (folic acid) and B6, and protection against coronary disease. It suggested that eating more fruits, vegetables, and whole grains, or getting these B vitamins from supplements, is as important as quitting smoking, lowering cholesterol, and controlling blood pressure in preventing premature death from the nation's leading killer (reported in Rimm, E.B., W.C. Willett, F.B. Hu, et al. "Folate and vitamin B6 from diet and supplements in relation to risk of coronary heart disease among women." *JAMA* 279:359–364 [1998]).

B vitamins are also known to be essential for breaking down carbohydrates into glucose (this provides energy for the body), for breaking down fats and proteins (which aids the normal functioning of the nervous system), and for muscle tone in the stomach and intestinal tract. They are also important in maintaining the health of skin, hair, eyes, mouth, liver, and more.

Vitamin B1: Thiamine

Casimir Funk discovered B1 in 1912. Also known as thiamine, it converts carbohydrates and fats into energy. It also helps prevent the buildup of toxic byproducts of this metabolism, which could otherwise damage the heart and nervous system. All B vitamins are involved in the process of converting food into energy, but thiamine plays a unique role, helping the brain and nervous system absorb enough glucose. Without thiamine, we become forgetful, depressed, tired, and apathetic. Good food sources of thiamine are Brazil nuts, sprouted seeds, sprouted beans, and germinated brown rice.

Vitamin B1 Reveals Another Synthetics Danger

In one experiment published in the journal *Nature* in 1939, authored by Dr. Barnett Sure, synthetic vitamin B1 (thiamine) was shown to render 100 percent of a group of pigs sterile—a significant finding.

If they knew that synthetic vitamin B1 was harmful to animals this many years ago, why did manufacturers continue to produce these and other synthetic supplements? The answer is that the drug companies that make synthetic vitamins have always promoted them as "natural" and safe, and the public (along with their so-called protectors, the federal government) has not questioned their contentions. Unfortunately, in our culture a drug is rarely labeled as dangerous until there is the potential for addiction or overdose demonstrated by illness and death statistics.

Synthetic thiamine is found in fortified breads, cereals, pasta, whole grains, dried beans, peas, and soybeans. Naturally occurring forms are found in fruits and vegetables. Thiamine is essential for brain and immune-cell function.

Vitamin B2: Riboflavin

D.T. Smith and E.G. Hendrick discovered B2, also known as riboflavin, in 1926.

Riboflavin, called vitamin B2, breaks down carbohydrates, fats, and proteins, and converts them into energy. B2 is significant in the maintenance of the skin and mucous membranes, the cornea of the eye, for nerve sheaths, and for red blood cell production. Riboflavin also acts as a coenzyme for oxidation-reduction reactions throughout the body, and works with other vitamins in the B complex to process calories from carbohydrates, protein, and fat. Because oxidation reactions cause damage to our cells, minimizing them can help us overcome many diseases.

Without riboflavin and other B vitamins, our body fails to release energy from protein, fat, and carbohydrates during metabolism. Riboflavin supports our immune system by keeping the mucous membranes that line the respiratory and digestive systems healthy. Riboflavin may also help make antibodies for fighting off infections and help to preserve the integrity of the nervous system, eyes, skin, nails, and hair. There is evidence that older people with high levels of riboflavin do better on memory tests. Both niacin (B3) and pyridoxine (B6) need riboflavin to function properly. Riboflavin activates pyridoxine and is essential for the conversion of tryptophan, a neurotransmitter often associated with nerve "calming" into niacin. This means that a deficiency in riboflavin can cause malabsorption of and deficiencies in other vitamins such as tryptophan and niacin.

Vitamin B3: Niacin

Vitamin B3, also known as niacin, is needed for more than 50 body processes. Like all the B-complex vitamins, it is important for release of energy from carbohydrates and fats, the metabolism of proteins, the creation of certain hormones, and assisting in the formation of red blood cells.

Although niacin is a crucial factor in energy production, it may not be the first reason why people need it. Niacin helps balance cholesterol levels. It makes enzymes that help cells turn carbohydrates into energy. The coenzymes NAD and NADP are essential for utilizing the metabolic energy of foods. The important role of niacin in energy production is that it helps control blood-glucose levels. Niacin is useful in the production of fatty acids, promotes appetite, aids in digestion, and supports healthy skin and nerves. It assists in the breakdown of proteins and fats and in the formation of red blood cells, and has been used successfully to increase blood flow.

American Conrad Elvehjem discovered vitamin B3 in 1937. It is found naturally in fresh water algae, sea vegetables, raw sprouted nuts, and other sprouts. Legumes also supply some niacin. Like all the B-complex vitamins, it is important for converting calories from protein, fat, and carbohydrates into energy. Additionally, it helps the digestive system function.

Vitamin B5: Pantothenic Acid

Pantothenic acid is found throughout living cells in the form of coenzyme A (CoA), which is vital to numerous biological reactions. Your body needs pantothenic acid to convert food (fat, carbohydrates, and proteins) into energy. It also helps in healing wounds. Administration of pantothenic acid orally and the application of pantothenol ointment to the skin have been shown to accelerate the closure of skin wounds and increase the strength of scar tissue.

Pantothenic acid is needed to make two crucial coenzymes: coenzyme A (CoA) and acyl carrier protein (ACP). CoA is required for the synthesis of essential fats, cholesterol, and steroid hormones, as well as the synthesis of the neurotransmitter acetylcholine and the hormone melatonin. It is also used by the liver for the metabolism of a number of toxins. The acyl carrier protein (ACP), like CoA, is required for the synthesis of fatty acids. Fatty acids are a component of lipids, which are fat molecules essential for normal physiological function. These enzymes help you use fats and carbohydrates to make energy. You also need them for making some important hormones, in the production of healthy red blood cells, and for making vitamin D.

Pantothenic acid and biotin are found in sprouted whole-grain cereals and legumes, broccoli and broccoli sprouts, sweet potatoes, and other vegetables in the cabbage family.

Vitamin B6: Pyridoxine

Paul Gyorgy discovered vitamin B6 in 1934, and readily understood this element to be a cell builder and cell stimulant.

There are currently six known forms of vitamin B6: pyridoxal (PL), pyridoxine (PN), pyridoxamine (PM), and their phosphate derivatives: pyridoxal 5'-phosphate (PLP), pyridoxine 5'-phosphate (PNP), and pridoxamine 5'-phospate (PNP). PLP is the active coenzyme form, and seems to be of the most importance in human metabolism. However, pyridoxine (PN) is the most common form of vitamin B6. With less than 2 mg a day of vitamin B6, your body is able to make more than 60 different known enzymes. B6 helps your immune system function and keeps your red blood cells strong while helping your nerves communicate with the rest of your body. It also is useful for preventing cramping during menstrual cycles. This is commonly found in green vegetables, most grains, sunflower green sprouts, and sea vegetables.

Vitamin B7: Biotin

Biotin is water soluble and generally classified as a B-complex vitamin. After the initial discovery of biotin, nearly 40 years of research was required to establish it as a vitamin fraction and categorize it within the B-vitamins section. Studies have shown biotin may help create healthy hair and prevent brittle nails, and is required to properly metabolize fats and amino acids. Its most healthy forms can be found in sprouted grains, adzuki sprouts, and whole-grain rice.

Vitamin B9: Folic Acid

Folates are a group of compounds derived from folic acid. They are required for cell division and the formation of DNA (the body's genetic blueprint) and RNA (which transports DNA data within the cell), and for protein synthesis. Folate is also vital for reproduction and for the development of the iron-containing protein in hemoglobin needed to make red blood cells. The terms *folic acid* and *folate* are often used interchangeably for this water-soluble B-complex vitamin. Folic acid is the form most often used in synthetic vitamin supplements and fortified foods. Naturally occurring folates are found in foods as well as in metabolically active forms in the human body.

We need folic acid to build muscles and to keep the body strong and in good repair. Folic acid is one of the most essential elements in the body to help replace failing body cells with new ones. It is especially important for reproducing cells that wear out and divide rapidly, such as red blood cells, skin cells, and the cells that line the small intestine.

Folic acid (also known as folate) is one of the B-complex vitamins that is known to work with vitamin B12 and vitamin C to break down proteins and for the formation of hemoglobin (a compound in red blood cells essential for transferring oxygen and carbon dioxide). In the past few years we have learned that folic acid helps to prevent birth defects and heart disease, and may even help to prevent cancer. The evidence is so convincing that since 1998 many common grain products, including bread, cereal, pasta, and rice, have been fortified with folic acid in an attempt to replace what has been removed in the manufacturing process, but natural folic acid is available in all sprouted grains and in fresh, leafy vegetables. Consuming sprouted and germinated grains can prevent all of these disorders.

Folate deficiency is one of the most common nutrient deficiencies and can result in megaloblastic anemia, which is characterized by a reduced number of red blood cells. Side effects of anemia include weakness, fatigue, headache, irritability, difficulty concentrating, and shortness of breath.

Vitamin B12: Cobalamin

Vitamin B12 is a soil-based microorganism and the best-known and most complex of all the known B vitamin family. It is unique in that it contains a metal ion, cobalt. For this reason, cobalamin is the term used to refer to compounds having B12 activity. Methylcobalamin and 5-deoxyadenosyl cobalamin are some of the forms of vitamin B12 used in the human body. The form of cobalamin used in most synthetic supplements is called cyanocobalamin. Cobalamin is known to help keep red blood cells healthy.

Studies we have conducted at Hippocrates on B12 deficits found that well more than half the general population lacks an adequate store of this vital nutrient. When you lack this nutrient and red blood cells cannot carry oxygen and nutrients through your body, you may develop pernicious anemia. Your brain becomes the first target when B12 is in deficit, with memory loss and even Alzheimer's as a consequence. Vitamin B12 is also integral to the making of DNA, RNA, and myelin, the white sheath protecting nerve fibers. Your nervous system also requires B12, and without it, begins to erode.

All cells, not just your red blood cells, need B12 to grow and divide properly. This includes the white blood cells required for a healthy immune system. Cobalamin helps maintain the health of the body's nerve sheath, the fatty layer that surrounds the nerve cells and protects healthy nerve function. Working with the other B vitamins, including pyridoxine and folic acid, B12 helps turn the carbohydrates, fats, and proteins in food into cellular energy. Rice sprouts and wheat grass are naturally high in the whole B vitamin complex, yet alone do not supply enough of it. We recommend full-spectrum extracts of wheat and rice, which contain high-quality natural sources of the B vitamin complex combined with a bacterial living form of B12 supplement.

Vitamin B12 is found in freshwater algae and sea vegetables. Yet it is necessary for all of us to ingest a bacterial supplemental form on a daily basis; it must be a naturally occurring source of the vitamin. Animal food consumption does not provide a digestible and complete form of this common essential nutrient.

Vitamin C's Crucial Health Role

Once again, you may not want to believe it, but here is the ugly truth about vitamin C, one of the most popular vitamin supplements sold in the world today: Rather than bolstering your body's defenses against the common cold and other maladies, once it is in your body it becomes no more than just another toxin that your organs and immune system must flush out of your system. That is because the vast majority of vitamin C sold and consumed in the world is synthetic.

Vitamin C is one of the most unstable vitamins, easily destroyed by oxidation through exposure to light or heat. Ascorbic acid is only the "antioxidant wrapper" portion of vitamin C, but this is the form most often sold to consumers. In and of itself, ascorbic acid is not able to supply your body with this essential nutrient in a complete form. Ascorbic acid protects the functional parts of the vitamin from rapid oxidation or breakdown. Vitamin C is vital for healing infections, wounds, and burns, and for the formation of collagen, a protein essential for healthy skin, bones, cartilage, teeth, and gums.

Vitamin C also helps to produce the neurotransmitters noradrenaline (which regulates blood flow) and serotonin (which promotes sleep as well as calm, joyful, and productive states of mind). Vitamin C also improves iron uptake because the iron present in many plant foods (known as non-haem iron) is absorbed more efficiently when these foods are accompanied by vitamin C–rich foods or a whole-food-based vitamin C supplement. In addition to ascorbic acid, real vitamin C includes mineral cofactors and the bioflavonoids hesperidin, rutin, quercitin, and tannin along with other naturally occurring components. If any one of these components is missing, there is no vitamin C activity, resulting in inadequate supplementation that could result in any number of such deficiency-related illnesses as bleeding, premature aging of organs including the skin, nerve damage, loss of sexual function, and impaired eyesight.

Most ascorbic acid (more than 95 percent) is just a chemical copy of naturally occurring ascorbic acid, which itself is still only a fraction of the actual whole vitamin C. Real vitamin C can only come from a complete full-spectrum whole food matrix; fractionated chemical ascorbic acid, on the other hand, is just another toxin to your body. Most ascorbic acid, manufactured by a few of the world's largest drug manufacturers, is usually fermented from cornstarch, corn sugar, and volatile acids. Most U.S. vitamin manufacturing companies buy the bulk ascorbic acid from these facilities then make their own formulations, labels, and claims, even though it likely originated from the same manufacturer. All of them, however, have the same ill effects.

How Synthetics Came About (The Grave History)

As you know, in 1747, Scottish naval surgeon James Lind discovered, while sailing with the English fleet, that a nutrient in citrus fruits (now known to be vitamin C) prevented scurvy. His theory and paper were not accepted by naval authorities until much later. The English government and military, as well as the rest of the population, took food for granted, not thinking of it as medicine. In fact, it took another 100 years before science developed to the point that it could begin to research and comprehend food's nutritional benefits. Progress in science was slow during those times; technological developments in chemistry and most sciences did not heat up until the beginning of the 20th century. In 1912, vitamin C was rediscovered and identified by Norwegians A. Hoist and T. Froelich, and in 1935 it became the first vitamin to be artificially synthesized by a process invented by Dr. Tadeusz Reichstein of the Swiss Institute of Technology in Zurich.

In 1932, Hungarian biochemist Albert Szent-Györgyi, MD, PhD, isolated a substance he called hexuronic acid (later known as ascorbic acid) from the adrenal glands. At around the same time, W.A. Waugh and Charles King isolated a vitamin from lemon and showed that it was nearly identical to hexuronic acid. Szent-Györgyi, who received the 1937 Nobel Prize for his discovery of vitamin C and the flavonoids, may have been the first scientist to raise the vitamin consciousness of his colleagues. In his letters on oxidation, published in 1939, Szent-Györgyi wrote:

> I had a letter from an Austrian colleague who was suffer-
> ing from a severe hemorrhagic diathesis [bleeding capil-
> laries]. He wanted to try ascorbic acid for his condition.
> Possessing at that time no sufficient quantities of crys-
> talline ascorbic acid, I sent him a preparation of pa-
> prika that contained much ascorbic acid and the man
> was cured by it. Later with my friend, St. Rusznyak, we
> tried to produce the same therapeutic effect in similar
> conditions with pure [laboratory-produced] ascorbic
> acid, but we obtained no response. It was evident that
> the action of paprika was due to some other [naturally
> occurring] substance(s) in this plant.

Szent-Györgyi realized that naturally occurring vitamin C contained additional factors, unknown at the time, which synergized and increased the potency of the vitamin. He was able through this discovery to help those who were unable to receive benefits from the isolated ascorbic acid or synthetic vitamin C. Szent-Györgyi found that he could never heal scurvy with isolated ascorbic acid itself. He realized, however, that he could always eliminate scurvy with the "matrix" vitamin C found in simple foods. He had arrived at the same conclusion as the English surgeon James Lind had 200 years earlier: other factors had to be present in order for vitamin C activity to take place. He eventually revealed another member of the vitamin C complex, the bioflavonoid rutin.

As Drs. Royal Lee and Szent-Györgyi both came to understand, all of the factors in the vitamin C complex—ascorbic acid, rutin, and additional elements—were synergists: cofactors that together sparked the functional interdependence of biologically related nutrient factors. In 1939, Szent-Györgyi gave a series of guest lectures at Vanderbilt University Medical School in Nashville, Tennessee, in which he said that it was impossible to predict how many more vitamins would be discovered. He was deeply interested in the difference between the "minimum daily doses" of vitamins needed to prevent deficiency diseases and optimal doses.

When Dr. Szent-Györgyi first isolated ascorbic acid as an antidote for scurvy, this isolate did not completely heal scurvy, but simply lessened its symptoms. Later when vitamin C in the natural form taken from peppers was used, it eradicated scurvy completely. The difference was that ascorbic acid in food is always found along with a class of compounds called bioflavonoids, which, based on Szent-Györgyi's findings, are necessary as a scurvy relief.

Once again, bear in mind that in nature vitamins are never isolated in pure crystalline states as are synthetic vitamins. They are always found in combination with other naturally occurring and synergistic factors that enable them to function correctly. These associated factors include proteins, trace elements, enzymes, hormones, phytonutrients, minerals, and other substances in a full nutrient complex. So, as with all vitamins and nutrients, for maximum benefit it is better to use an authentic full-spectrum food source of vitamin C than a fractional part of vitamin C. You might consider the Amla berry, a common fruit in India and parts of China, as it contains one of the highest concentrations of naturally occurring vitamin C in nature, much higher than oranges, Acerola cherries, limes, or any other ripe fruit.

Following are a few of the thousands of supporting comments that have accumulated throughout the decades extolling complete vitamin C as superior to ascorbic acid for protection of your body:

⊘ "It was demonstrated that guinea pigs, fed vitamin C–free diets, could be more thoroughly protected against infections with pneumococci [a bacteria related to pneumonia] by lemon juice or orange juice than by

pure ascorbic acid [alone]. (Stepp, W., J. Kuhnau, and
J. Schroeder, *The Vitamins and Their Clinical
Applications* [*Die Vitamine und ihre luisdhe Anwendung*]
Ferdinand Enke, Stuttgart, Germany, 1936)

⊘ Professor Lesne believes that the effect of natural
vitamins is superior to that of the artificial ones. For
instance, "The treatment of scurvy by giving 50 cc of
lemon juice containing 25 mg of ascorbic acid
produces quicker results than 25 mg of ascorbic acid
[alone] administered as a medicament." (*Journal of the
American Medical Assoc.* 118, 6:475, Feb. 7, 1942)

Bioflavonoids, also known as flavonoids, are a group of beneficial
phytochemicals. In addition to being antioxidants, they promote arte-
rial health (quercetin), hormonal balance (isoflavones), and the health
of the retina (anthoycyanosides). Bioflavonoids, which are always found
as part of the naturally occurring vitamin C matrix, are the natural
pigments in fruits and vegetables. Researchers have reported more
than 800 different bioflavonoids. Most are the yellow, orange, or brown
pigments found in fruits and vegetables. Some researchers believe that
bioflavonoids, also referred to as vitamin P, help maintain capillaries,
the microscopic blood vessels in the body that allow oxygen, hormones,
nutrients, and antibodies to pass from the body's bloodstream into
individual cells. If capillary walls are too fragile, they will allow blood to
drain out of the vessels and into the cells. The result of this is easy
bruising, brain and retinal hemorrhages, bleeding gums, and other
abnormalities.

Bioflavonoids have been shown to aid in the clotting of blood.
This can be helpful in treating phlebitis and other clotting deficiencies
such as hemochromatosis. Many bioflavonoids prevent the cellular
damage caused by free radicals, the unstable molecules formed when
the body burns oxygen. Some reports show that bioflavonoids enhance
the antioxidant action of certain nutrients as well.

Researchers have discovered that ascorbic acid is credited with
some of the functions that actually come from bioflavonoids.

The critical point here is that ascorbic acid and bioflavonoids work
together to enhance the immune system. Many laboratory studies show

how bioflavonoids stop or slow the growth of malignant cells and protect against cancer-causing substances invading the heart and blood cells. Bioflavonoids also act as natural antibiotics, destroying bacteria present in food, which often cause food-borne infections. Bioflavonoids are also now being studied for general medical uses such as preventing bruising and bleeding abnormalities.

Other naturally occurring nutrients associated with whole vitamin C are tannins and ellagic acid. Tannins are excellent antioxidants, now being promoted by the health industry. Tannins, often recognized as pigments, are flavonoid-type compounds that have an action similar to bioflavonoids. High tannin tea has been shown to reduce the need for blood removal from people with iron overload, or hemochromatosis. Hemochromatosis is a genetic defect that causes uncontrolled absorption of iron. Affecting one person in 200, iron overload is a major factor in congestive heart failure, a rapidly growing burden on the healthcare system.

Tannins, also called catechins, which are polyphenols, appear to be one of the most potent therapeutic plant-derived, naturally occurring chemicals. Aside from their antiseptic and antioxidant properties, they are able to form complexes with other molecules to detoxify the system.

Ellagic acid is a compound found in certain fruits such as red raspberries and Amla berries. Research in cell cultures and lab animals has found that ellagic acid may slow the growth of some tumors caused by certain carcinogens. Although this is promising, at this time there is no reliable evidence from human studies showing that ellagic acid in any form can prevent or treat cancer. Further research is needed to determine what benefits it may have. Professor Gary Stoner from Ohio State University, referring specially to dark (black and blue) raspberries, registered a patent on June 23, 2005, relating to fighting cancers and their metastases with ellagic acid.

It is the ellagitannins that are present in red raspberries and other fruits such as Amla or Indian gooseberry. Ellagic acid may act as a scavenger to "bind" cancer-causing chemicals, rendering them inactive. It appears to disarm chemicals that cause mutations in bacteria. In addition, ellagic acid may help prevent binding of carcinogens to

DNA and reduce the incidence of cancer in cultured human cells exposed to these toxins.

More Ways to Distinguish Natural From Synthetic

A couple of dramatic methods for showing the difference between a natural vitamin and a synthetic vitamin are the use of chromatograms and energy photographs. Chromatagrams are made by mixing water with the dry vitamin material and then spreading it on a sheet of absorbent paper through a blotting process to show the symmetrical designs of natural substances versus the less symmetrical designs of synthetic substances. (See page 41 for an example of chromatograms.)

Energy photographs or videos designed to measure the electromagnetic field of a substance are made by taking any object and passing an electrical current through it while using an exposure photographic technique that produces an image of the electrical current both inside and around the object. This image is the closest measure we have for "seeing" what scientists call an electromagnetic field.

In the last 25 years, we have discovered that sub-particles occupy the radius of minerals and trace minerals and act as conduits to and from larger nutrients. Together they fulfill the task of complete absorption and proper function. When processing or cooking foods and whole-food supplements, these sub-particles are destroyed, thereby significantly reducing both the potency and function of the remaining molecule. The foods and supplements are essentially stripped of their nutritive value, rendering them dead and denatured.

This is a cutting-edge scientific way to illustrate the difference between whole and synthetic vitamins. It can be an eye-opening experience for those who believe in the magnificence and symmetry of nature and in the life force surrounding all living organisms, including living foods. There are forces in nature that are necessary for life but cannot be re-created in a lab. The study of these forces, to this day, remains almost exclusively the domain of physical science and physicists rather than that of the biological sciences (doctors, nutritionists, chemists, and biologists.) Until this gap between the sciences is bridged, food science will continue to lag behind in its application of this fundamental universal principle of the natural world.

Fortunately, a growing number of professionals from the biological community are bridging this gap and making important contributions in the area of health sciences. In our collective opinion, nothing could have more significance or as great an impact on the health of the planet and its people than the understanding and adoption of whole-food, plant-based nutrition. For this to happen, however, we must stand together as a global community and insist on the universal application of truly natural food principles. Truly natural is *always* better when it comes to nutrition.

Following is an energy photograph of Amla-C, a naturally occurring, food-derived vitamin C tablet illustrating a strong bio-energy field.

Here are some results of a Kirlian photography study indicating the electromagnetic field surrounding natural Amla berry vitamin C and synthesized ascorbic acid vitamin C materials. (Courtesy of Vedic Science Institute, Cobb, California, 1994).

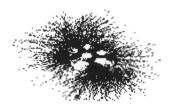

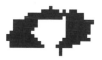

Amla C Sample.   *Other Vitamin C Sample*
                                          (Ascorbic Acid).

It is quite easy to see the difference in vital energy that each material offers.

A true and natural vitamin C is a complex matrix of naturally occurring compounds derived from fruit or some other food that not only contains the compound ascorbic acid but also contains other necessary components of the vitamin C matrix such as flavonoids like hesperin or rutin, tannins, and other factors, some of which may still be unknown.

Ascorbic acid ($C6H806$) is *not* vitamin C. It is a chemical fraction—an isolated part—of what could be a real (Naturally Occurring

Standard—NOS) vitamin C. In this form it is always and only synthetic. In studies carried out on food-based vitamin C, research has concluded that it acts very differently than synthetic vitamin C. The food-based C is more slowly absorbed and has higher bioavailability. One long-term study by J.A. Vinson, unpublished but titled "Bioavailability of Vitamin C" in 1991, showed the food-based citrus extract vitamin C to be up to 12 times more bioavailable than ascorbic acid.

This means that more of the vitamin is absorbed into the plasma, and it is retained substantially longer with less excreted in urine. Therefore, it is of higher overall value to our bodies.

Your Teeth and Vitamin C

Although a great deal of consumer information cautions against chewing large amounts of ascorbic acid because of its erosive effects on tooth enamel, other scientific studies have addressed this issue differently. One study found that dissolving a 500 mg chewable vitamin C tablet in one's mouth caused enamel erosion. But, chewable vitamin C tablets of 250 mg and 60 mg did not produce enough acidity to cause enamel erosion.

Although some chewable tablets are buffered with sodium, the researchers felt that the sodium might be of insufficient quantity to prevent dental erosion (reported in Hays, G.L., et al., "Salivary pH while dissolving vitamin C-containing tablets," *American Journal of Dentistry* 5:269–271 [1992]). Because the application of vitamin C directly to the teeth and gums has no known therapeutic value, they recommended swallowing vitamin C tablets instead of chewing them. Some health advisors recommend rinsing the mouth with water once the ascorbic acid tablet is taken orally so that tooth enamel is not dissolved by the synthetic vitamin C (ascorbic acid). It is important to point out that all of these tests were done with lab-derived vitamin C, and the higher the amount the greater the problem identified.

Please remember that vitamin C is found in citrus fruits and their juices, strawberries, cantaloupes, tomatoes, broccoli, sweet potatoes, sprouts, and turnip greens and other greens. Most other fruits and vegetables contain some vitamin C. Other sources include black currants, clover, radish, and chickpea sprouts, guava, kiwi fruit, and red peppers.

CHAPTER 7

MINERALS IMPORTANT TO GOOD HEALTH

As you might imagine, the debate about taking naturally occurring mineral supplements from food sources versus synthetic mineral supplements made from non-living sources mirrors the natural-vitamin-versus-synthetic-vitamin controversy that is the dominant theme of this book.

At least 16 minerals have been identified as essential to human growth and reproduction. Macro-minerals such as calcium, magnesium, sodium, and potassium are required in comparatively large quantities, whereas micro-minerals such as iron and zinc, selenium, manganese, and iodine are necessary in much smaller amounts, though all remain important to our health.

Our mineral levels derived from foods are dependent on the levels of minerals present in the soils where the crops were grown. As you know from previous chapters of this book, we simply are not getting adequate supplies of minerals from our food crops unless the crops are organically grown in soils that have been revitalized with mineral content.

It is also important to note that various nutrients affect the body's ability to absorb minerals. Vitamin D, for example, is necessary for the uptake of calcium. Vitamin C is necessary for the absorption of iron, particularly iron found in plant foods. Copper is necessary for vitamin C activity. Mineral deficiencies also cause vitamin deficiencies, and worldwide we are seeing mineral deficiencies becoming a well-documented result of systematic soil depletion.

The body can maintain its own mineral balance throughout short periods. If the intake of minerals is low, it draws from stores in the muscles, the liver, and bones. If a mineral intake is too high, excesses are usually excreted so that there is little danger of the body being harmed, except by the use of synthetic supplements. Minerals aid in development of our bone structure, metabolic reactions, cell membrane transport of nutrients, muscle movement, and as part of the elements of blood and enzymes.

Minerals used in the body are classified as:

1. Macro-minerals, or the main minerals such as calcium, phosphorus, magnesium, potassium, sulfur, chloride, and sodium.

2. Trace minerals, such as iron, zinc, copper, iodine, fluoride, chromium, selenium, manganese, and molybdenum.

Other trace minerals include bromide, cadmium, vanadium, tin, nickel, aluminum, silicon, and many others. Although minerals are of vital importance, they make up only about 4 percent of your body's weight. All of the trace elements account for only about .01 percent of total body weight.

Minerals are vitally important nutrients that must be ingested on a regular basis in food or supplement form to maintain proper body function.

As with the controversy over synthetic versus natural vitamins, there is a controversy about the use of inorganic versus organic minerals. This controversy may be less pronounced than the natural and synthetic vitamin controversy, but it is still important to consider natural, organic mineral use for optimal health and longevity.

What is the difference between "organic" plant-based minerals and "non-organic" minerals?

Organic minerals are those derived from plant-based foods such as vegetables and botanicals. Organic minerals are received by consuming plant food. Their root systems convert rock-solid non-organic minerals into useable organic ones. The word *organic* is often misused by referring to a mineral or a specific chemical compound rather than a "living" entity, and that creates a lot of confusion.

As we have said, "organic" chemistry defines many toxic and poisonous compounds as organic, so the use of the word itself is problematic. It is clearer to refer to minerals as either *naturally occurring* in foods or *not naturally occurring*. Using the term *naturally occurring* is how we distinguish between natural and unnatural vitamins, so the same standard applies to minerals. These are the standards that we recommend to the food and supplement community because it eliminates any confusion concerning the issue of organic and non-organic minerals.

Minerals from food sources contain many cofactors such as enzymes, vitamins, hormones, oxygen, phytonutrients, enzymes, and other yet unknown elements.

As with vitamins, nature does not make isolated, individual minerals in foods without cofactors. All the naturally occurring minerals in food sources are naturally chelated (broken down to a digestible form) compounds that are bound to other nutrient factors such as other minerals, vitamins, hormones, enzymes, oxygen, and phytonutrient compounds that are in the food source itself. For example, when an alfalfa plant absorbs calcium carbonate from the soil, that calcium is metabolized and transformed through the plant's complex chemical "factory" into calcium phytate or other organic calcium compounds. In addition, other vitamins, mineral, and nutritional factors may have been united with the calcium phytate to form a unique source of naturally occurring calcium complex.

Botanicals have the ability to transmute compounds and nutritional factors into a useful, complex nutrient matrix such as a vitamin or a specialized protein. The naturally occurring minerals found in foods are "complexed" and pre-metabolized, making them more nutritionally useful and bioavailable than non-organic, non-food forms of minerals, which often accumulate in the body and cause calcium and mineral deposits as well as hardening of the arteries.

Calcium from food sources is more assimilable and bioavailable than calcium from rocks, sediments, and other non-organic mineral sources. Non-organic minerals are not formed by fresh, living matter and contain no vital carbon compounds. As do all organic minerals, organic calcium materials contain carbon that was once a part of, or produced or metabolized by, living plants or animals.

Calcium

Calcium is responsible for the construction, formation, and maintenance of bone and teeth. This function helps reduce the occurrence of osteoporosis. It is also a vital component in blood clotting systems and wound healing, and helps to control blood pressure, nerve transmission, and release of neurotransmitters. It is an essential component in the production of enzymes and hormones regulating digestion, energy, and fat metabolism. It helps transport ions (electrically charged particles) across the cell membranes and is essential for muscle contraction. Calcium assists in maintaining all cells and connective tissues in the body.

When the body needs more calcium than is supplied through diet, it withdraws it from the bones. This unfortunate but necessary biochemical activity frequently results in conditions such as osteoporosis and osteoarthritis, fractures, and so on. Foods that contain oxalic acid, in particular spinach and rhubarb, can prevent the absorption of calcium. The consumption of meat and dairy products has been shown to rob the minerals from bones, thereby weakening them and subjecting them to many diseases and conditions from fractures, arthritis, and osteoporosis. The United States has some of the world's highest rates of osteoporosis, and, not coincidentally, we consume equally high rates of dairy products. This is also true in the Nordic countries of Finland, Sweden, and Norway. If dairy products (cheese, milk, butter, and so on) were good sources of calcium, we would not have such high rates of these disorders.

Supplements are used to treat muscle cramps as well as problems of the back and bones related to improper aging, such as arthritis, rheumatism, and osteoporosis (the loss of bony tissue that results in brittle bones, particularly prevalent among post-menopausal women). These problems are in fact more an indication of improper living throughout a long period of time. Calcium deficiency often follows vitamin D deficiencies and can lead to rickets in children. Typical symptoms of rickets are bowlegs, knock-knees, and pigeon chests, all caused by softening of the bones. In adults, calcium deficiency can cause osteomalacia, characterized by aching bones, muscle spasms, and curvature of the spine.

Most calcium supplementation today is derived from calcium carbonate, which is found in chalk, oyster shells, coral rock sediments, eggshells, and other non-organic sediments and non-living mineral sources. Calcium from these sources is *not* an organic, naturally occurring food ingredient, and despite how it is marketed to consumers, it does not fulfill our nutritional needs.

It is a challenge to find a real and substantial vegetable source of calcium supplementation derived from food. (See Appendix A of this book for a few recommended sources of vegetable calcium supplementation.)

Calcium is the most abundant mineral in the body. The average male has about 3 pounds of calcium, the average female about 2 pounds. Most (99 percent) calcium is found in bones and teeth (according to the National Research Council, 1989; Whitney et al., 1996) with the remaining 1 percent in the soft tissues and watery parts of the body where calcium helps to regulate normal organ processes.

When blood calcium levels drop, the body can borrow from its skeletal stores and return calcium to bones as needed. A constant supply of calcium is necessary throughout our lifetime, but is especially important during phases of growth, pregnancy, and lactation. About 10 to 40 percent of dietary calcium is absorbed in the small intestine.

The level of calcium absorption from dietary sources drops in post-menopausal women. The body will absorb more calcium if there is a deficiency.

Factors that improve calcium absorption include adequate amounts of protein, magnesium, phosphorous, and vitamin D. Conditions that reduce calcium absorption include high or excessive intakes of oxalates and phytates, found in foods such as cooked spinach. Consumption of alcohol, coffee, sugar, or medications such as diuretics, tetracycline, and aluminum-containing antacids, as well as stress, reduces the absorption of calcium and other minerals.

Lack of exercise reduces calcium absorption as well as causing an increase in calcium losses. A lifestyle of immobility also leads to calcium deficiency. Calcium deficiency increases the risk of bone disorders such as osteoporosis.

Naturally occurring sources of calcium include dark green leafy vegetables, sprouted beans, pea greens, corn sprouts, green juice, and some botanicals. There is a high level of naturally occurring vegetable calcium available in Terminalia arjuna (known as "Arjuna" herb), a traditional medicinal botanical grown in Asia. Some extracts of this herb are specifically offered as calcium supplements.

Magnesium

An important constituent of bone is magnesium, which assists in transmitting nerve impulses; it is also important for muscle contraction. It acts as an essential cofactor for many enzymes, which function properly only when magnesium is present. Two such enzymes, 97 co-carboxylase and coenzyme A97, are involved in extracting energy from food. Mild magnesium deficiency is more common than previously recognized, especially in people suffering from diabetes, malabsorption syndromes, celiac disease, and some forms of kidney disease. Those on anti-coagulants also suffer magnesium deficiencies.

Magnesium deficiency is a cause of cardiac arrhythmia (irregular heartbeat) and has been linked to premenstrual syndrome (PMS). Magnesium is found naturally in dark green leafy vegetables, nuts and seeds, and most sprouts, as well as whole grains, sprouted beans and peas, and some botanicals such as Terminalia arjuna.

Phosphorus

Phosphorus compounds (phosphates) are major constituents in the tissues of all plant and animal cells. As much as 80 percent of the body's phosphorus is found in our bones and teeth.

The process of creating bone tissue is known as calcification, which involves large amounts of phosphate as well as calcium and may be more accurately called mineralization.

Phosphorus is essential to the release of energy in cells, and to the absorption and transportation of many nutrients. It also regulates the activity of proteins. The intake of phosphorus has an important influence on the body's calcium status: if there is too much phosphorus, calcium absorption may be reduced. High intakes of phosphorus increase the body's secretion of parathyroid hormone, which may upset the body's calcium balance by removing calcium from the bones. An excessive intake of phosphorus can also inhibit magnesium absorption.

Phosphorus in its natural, bioavailable state is abundant in sprouted beans and peas, blue-green algae, kelp, dulse, and other sea vegetables.

Potassium

Cells, nerves, and muscles do not function properly without potassium. It works with sodium to maintain the fluid and electrolyte balance in cells and tissues, to regulate blood pressure, and to maintain a normal heartbeat. It helps counteract the effects of excess sodium intake, such as edema (fluid retention) and high blood pressure. Potassium is also vital for the transmission of nerve impulses from the brain to every part of the body. It is therefore critical for proper functioning.

Blood potassium levels are carefully regulated by hormones, and any excess intake is normally excreted through the kidneys. Symptoms of excess potassium are lethargy, paralysis, and a slow heartbeat. Early signs of potassium deficiency are apathy, weakness, confusion, and excessive thirst.

Potassium is found in most plant foods, but especially good sources include avocados, nuts and seeds, sprouted whole grains, beans and peas, fresh ripe tomatoes and green juices, bananas, kiwis, and oranges.

Sodium Chloride (Salt)

Salt, or sodium chloride, was the first mineral identified and regularly used as part of our diets (though in its non- or inorganic form, it plays havoc), probably because it is easily detected by the taste buds. Sodium is a major component of all body fluids, and is largely responsible for determining the body's total water content. Together with potassium, it is a key substance in regulating the balance of body fluids. It controls the levels of electrolytes in blood plasma and helps to regulate nerve and muscle function. It is also the antiseptic in lymph fluid.

Because sodium is lost in significant amounts through sweat, people living in hot climates or who exercise strenuously can run a risk of a deficiency. One of the first symptoms is a cramp, which often affects the calf or leg muscles. A serious deficiency can lead to dehydration, causing low blood pressure, dryness of the mouth, and vomiting. High sodium intakes can lead to edema (fluid retention) and high blood pressure, leading to heart failure, strokes, or kidney failure.

Chloride

Chloride acts with potassium and sodium to maintain the body's fluid and electrolyte balance. The highest concentrations of chloride in the body are found in cerebrospinal fluid and in digestive juices in the stomach. The main dietary source of chloride is table salt (sodium chloride), but it is not advisable to consume any non-organic sodium such as table salt, crystal salt, sea salt, and so on; these sodium chloride–rich salts dehydrate the body and raise blood pressure. Consume organic sodium minerals through foods such as celery or sea vegetables in order to maintain healthy levels of chloride. When dietary intake is low, the kidneys can reabsorb chloride efficiently, so a dietary deficiency rarely occurs. Excessive chloride losses can occur in the same way as sodium loss: through sweating, diarrhea, and vomiting.

Trace Minerals You Need

Similar to the better-known macro-minerals, these micro- or trace minerals are stored primarily in your bone or muscle tissue. Even though we need these trace elements in much smaller doses, they still play crucial roles in facilitating physiological health. Generally speaking, if your body requires more than 100 milligrams each day, it is a mineral, but if less than 100 milligrams a day, it is a trace element.

Aluminum

Although most minerals pose little threat to health, aluminum may be an important exception. Trace amounts of the mineral are found in all living organisms. However, scientists are still not sure about its biological function in the body. The mineral makes up some 8 percent of the Earth's crust, yet plants—with the exception of tea—take up remarkably little of it from the soil.

In most cases the aluminum taken in by the human body is excreted rather than absorbed. There is a general belief in the scientific and medical community that excessive amounts of aluminum in the diet can cause brain damage and may exacerbate disorders such as Alzheimer's disease. This idea remains contentious; nonetheless, we recommend avoiding aluminum cookware, food wrappings, and food additives as a safeguard.

Aluminum is added to table salt to prevent the grains from sticking together. It is added to underarm deodorants to help prevent perspiration. Low levels of aluminum can also occur in tap water because aluminum sulphate is often used in its purification. Aluminum hydroxide is an ingredient in many antacid tablets used to treat indigestion, and the mineral may also be dissolved by acidic foods, such as tomato sauce, pickles, or stewed fruit that have been cooked in aluminum pans.

Chromium

An adequate supply of chromium is particularly important in a diabetic's diet as a vital link in the chain that makes glucose available to the body. Chromium increases the effectiveness of insulin by stimulating glucose uptake in cells. It also helps control levels of fat and cholesterol in the blood. A deficiency of the mineral can lead to high blood-cholesterol levels. Good sources of chromium include sprouted whole grains, hijiki and other sea vegetables, and sweet green peas.

Copper

A component of several enzymes, such as superoxide dismutase, which helps protect against free radical damage, copper is vital in forming connective tissue, which supports and separates organs and is found in tendons, bone, and cartilage. Copper is important for the growth of healthy bones and helps the body to absorb iron from food. A lack of copper can lead to iron-deficiency anemia because the mineral helps to make stored iron available for red blood cell production. Copper is also involved in the formation of melanin, the pigment that colors skin and hair.

Sprouted nuts and immune-building mushrooms such as maitake, shitake, and reishi are good vegetable sources of the mineral. Deficiency is rare, usually occurring only in premature babies—infants who are malnourished or who suffer from chronic diarrhea, or those with malabsorption problems. Copper deficiencies cause premature graying of hair, as well as joint and muscle pain.

Fluoride

Although a lack of fluoride can lead to childhood tooth decay, too much either in the diet or from other sources, such as swallowed toothpaste, tea, and fluoridated tap water, can cause fluorosis with its unsightly symptoms of mottled teeth with pitted enamel. Fluorosis may also cause excess bone formation, resulting in bones that are much denser than normal, but also less flexible, making them prone to fractures. Many health professionals believe that excess fluoride may be linked to forms of cancer (according to the article "Fluoride Linked to Bone Cancer in Boys," by Dr. C.W. Jameson, National Toxicology Program, Report on Carcinogens. Research Triangle Park, NC 27709, June 6, 2005, at *www.ewg.org/issues/fluoride/20050606/petition.php*).

Fluoride is not considered essential for life, but it does play a role in the maintenance of healthy bones: Fluoride combines with calcium to strengthen them. A deficiency, when associated with low intakes of calcium, may lead to osteoporosis.

Differing levels of fluoride occur naturally in soils and affect the amounts found in crops; most healthy organic vegetables grown in good soil contain fluoride. In many parts of the world, tea is the main source of dietary fluoride, as tea plants readily absorb the mineral from the soil.

Iodine

Sea vegetation, blue-green and green algae, and freshwater algae offer some of the best sources of iodine, which is also found in fruits, vegetables, and sprouted cereals. The amount of iodine in land vegetables depends on the amount of the mineral in the soil in which they are grown.

Iodine is needed to make thyroid hormones, which not only govern the rate and efficiency at which food is converted into energy, but also regulate physical and mental development.

Mild iodine deficiency leads to a slightly enlarged thyroid gland (or goiter), and is most likely to occur in women of reproductive age. Eating seaweed or sea vegetation supplements easily prevents the deficiency. Women with severe iodine deficiencies risk bearing children deficient in thyroid hormone; those children could, unless treated from birth with thyroxine, suffer from a form of retardation known as cretinism.

Iron

Hemoglobin, the pigment in red blood cells that carries oxygen around the body via the bloodstream, cannot be produced without iron. A shortage of this mineral quickly shows itself in breathlessness, as the heart pumps faster and the lungs try to increase the body's oxygen intake. Iron is also required for the manufacture of myoglobin, another pigment that stores oxygen in muscles.

Iron-containing enzymes assist in the conversion of beta-carotene (found in many deeply pigmented plant foods such as carrots, red peppers, apricots, and cantaloupes) into the active form of vitamin A. Other iron-containing enzymes are needed for the synthesis of DNA and RNA, and for the synthesis of collagen, which is essential for healthy skin, gums, teeth, cartilage, and bones.

Women, from the onset of monthly periods until menopause, need almost twice as much dietary iron as men. Lack of adequate dietary iron can result in iron deficiency anemia, with chronic infections of the ears, gums, and skin, excessive tiredness and lack of stamina, as well as a pale complexion. More of the iron from plant sources such as chickpeas, lentils, and seaweed, all deep green, fresh vegetables and sprouts, along with most sea vegetables, is absorbed if it is accompanied by food or drinks containing whole-food vitamin C.

Manganese

Like many micro-minerals, manganese has a broad range of functions. It is essential for activating enzyme systems involved in the synthesis of cartilage. It is also a constituent of certain enzymes involved in the protection of tissues from free radical damage. Manganese is necessary to both thyroid hormone and sex hormone production, and is important in manufacturing cholesterol and insulin. It is also needed for storing glucose in the liver and for healthy bone growth.

Manganese deficiency reduces fertility as well as white blood cell count. Prolonged deficiencies result in breakdowns of the organ and immune systems. Manganese is mostly found in sea- and freshwater algae, and fruits and vegetables.

Molybdenum

Molybdenum is essential to the enzymes involved in the production of DNA and RNA, and those involved in producing energy from fat and in releasing iron from the body's stores. Molybdenum is found in tooth enamel, and it is possible, according to research by Mark McCarty in *Health Benefits of Supplemental Nutrition*, that it helps prevent tooth decay. A deficiency reduces lifespan and weakens oral health.

Molybdenum is derived by consuming sprouted nuts, kelp, pollens, and most root vegetables.

Selenium

Selenium (an antioxidant mineral) is part of the enzyme glutathione peroxidase, which is involved in protecting body tissues from free radical damage.

Without this mineral, normal growth and fertility would not occur, the liver would not function normally, important hormone production would not take place, and the immune system would not fully function. Its presence in the body is essential for healthy hair and skin, and is needed to maintain normal eyesight. There is now evidence that selenium may help protect against prostate cancer. A selenium deficiency weakens the immune system, thereby predisposing the body to an array of diseases.

As with many other micro-minerals, selenium levels in food are related to the amount of selenium in the soil where food is grown. Selenium is found in plant foods such as citrus, whole grains, and Brazil nuts.

Sulfur

Sulfur is present in every cell of the body, and is especially concentrated in the skin, nails, and hair. Most sulfur in the body is obtained as part of the protein intake, as it is an integral part of the sulfur-containing amino acids cysteine and methionine. It is also a part of at least three B vitamins; thiamin, pantothenic acid, and biotin. Inorganic forms of the mineral—sulfide, sulfates, and sulfites—are not needed in the diet. Indeed, chemical sulfites, used to preserve the color of dried foods (such as apricots), may trigger asthma attacks in susceptible individuals. In its pure form sulfur acts as an antifungal and antibacterial agent, and is used in creams for treating skin disorders such as acne. Sulfur helps to reduce pain and arthritis conditions. A deficiency of sulfur increases the chance of infections and fungal disorders and promotes bone erosion.

Sulfur is found in cabbage, kale, Brussels sprouts, onions, garlic, and their sprouts.

Zinc

Zinc is an essential component of a wide range of enzymes. It is also necessary for maintaining and replicating genetic material (DNA and RNA), enabling the body to interpret its genetic information.

This mineral is vital for the normal growth of the body. Zinc plays an especially important role in the development of the ovaries and the testes, and a deficiency in childhood and adolescence impairs growth and sexual development. It is also needed for the efficient functioning of the immune system.

Indeed, zinc is so important to the immune system that even a mild deficiency can lead to an increased risk of infection. The mineral is therefore especially important to the elderly, who may be particularly vulnerable to a wide range of inflammatory concerns. Zinc is also necessary for a healthy appetite and assists in our ability to taste foods. A deficiency in zinc has been proven to increase the incidence of colds and flu, prostate illness, and premature graying and loss of hair.

Some good plant-derived sources of zinc include mung bean sprouts, pumpkin seeds, sesame seeds, sunflower seeds, wheat grass, and spelt sprouts.

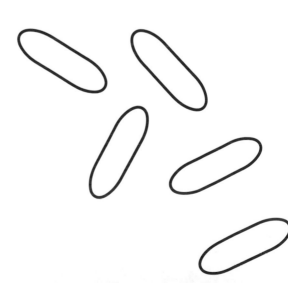

—— PART III ——

A NATURALLY OCCURRING STANDARD FOR SUPPLEMENTS

CHAPTER 8

WHAT ABOUT THE QUALITY OF DIRECT MARKET SUPPLEMENTS?

Though multi-level marketing (MLM) supplement sales currently make up just 20 percent or so of the entire supplements market, according to the industry journal *Nutrition Business*, countless numbers of consumers in the United States and elsewhere got their first introduction to the potential benefits of nutritional supplementation through direct contact with distributors working with network marketing companies (often called MLMs).

An estimated 14 million people in the United States today work part-time or full-time as direct marketers for about 1,200 direct marketing companies, with 50,000 joining each day. But the dropout rate for new direct marketers is high, by some estimates up to 98 percent within six months of joining. In spite of this high turnover, this form of distribution remains a relatively effective way to provide the general public with vitamin supplements, with the added bonus that this form of person-to-person contact can be a valuable way of educating people about the need for proper nutrition.

Comparing the quality of direct-marketed products versus those sold in traditional retail outlets is a question that has rarely been raised until now, but we consumers deserve to know that there are both similarities and differences that can and should impact our buying decisions.

In spite of claims of superior quality made by many direct marketing organizations, the majority of supplements sold by direct marketing organizations contain synthetic ingredients and adhere to the same basic production standards as the chemical supplements produced by conventional retail and pharmaceutical firms. As a result, they can suffer from the same limitations in quality. The majority of supplements we are speaking of, which is to say any non–Naturally Occurring Standard supplement, regardless of how they are distributed, tend to perpetuate a myth of quality that needs to be dispelled.

Be Wary of Inflated Claims

Marketing and advertising campaigns try to create a perception of quality and superiority of one brand of product over another, and so must engage in some degree of hype or even myth-making that can stretch or hide the truth. That is the inherent nature of the economic competition game. But unlike other categories of consumer products, those products that affect our health require special scrutiny so that hype and reality part ways in our decision-making.

The inadequate labeling laws currently in place, as discussed previously in this book, encourage some supplement sellers to stretch the boundaries of truth about the purity and effectiveness of their ingredients and products. Of course, many of these same supplement makers actually do believe their own hype, and not just for the convenience of financial gain, but because they have bought into—and have failed to question—a synthetics belief system that places the creations of the laboratory on a level equal to the creations of nature.

Federal laws prohibit employees of supplement retail stores from making medical claims or dispensing medical advice to customers about which particular products they should use to treat diseases or symptoms of disease. It is true that many retailers and their employees learn how to skirt these laws in a variety of ways, and the potential for the abuse of customer trust escalates sharply when direct marketing person-to-person contact comes into play.

In a direct marketing system, the emphasis is on product distributors recruiting more distributors to form networks so that sales profits are distributed both "downline" to associated distributors and "upline" to the parent corporation. The origins of this distribution concept can be traced back to 1959 and two young entrepreneurs who founded the Amway Corporation. They expanded on an idea developed in the 1930s by American businessman Carl Rehnborg, who produced food supplements and encouraged his friends to sell them on commission. His California Vitamin Corp. changed its name to Nutrilite Products in 1939, and within eight years it had 15,000 door-to-door sales agents who promoted the product using a booklet titled "How to Get Well and Stay Well."

This booklet claimed the supplement was effective in "almost every case" against asthma, allergies, irregular heartbeat, depression, and at least 30 other common maladies. It also implied that the supplement could treat heart disease, cancer, and every serious illness known to humankind. When the U.S. Food and Drug Administration brought legal action challenging these declarations, a federal court in 1951 issued a permanent injunction forbidding the company and its agents from making such unsubstantiated claims.

Most direct marketers today emphasize the illegality of making medical claims about supplement products, yet the words often fall on the deaf ears of enthusiastic distributors who have set sights instead on the promise of financial freedom. In truth, the majority of direct marketers are selling financial opportunity, even if they initially approach you about the quality of their product. This is part of the reason why the direct marketing industry has earned itself a less-than-favorable reputation throughout the years.

Many direct marketing companies also require their distributors to purchase product samples, or even require them to buy promotional and teaching materials such as CDs and DVDs, or they must pay for attendance at conferences and conventions. All of this contributes to pressure that distributors feel to recruit others into their network, even if they have to make exaggerated claims about profits that can be made and the effectiveness and value of the products being marketed.

An analysis of more than 100 direct marketing companies offering health-related products, mostly vitamins and other supplements, was conducted in 2003 by the National Council Against Health Fraud, which reached a series of conclusions:

⊘ Every one of the multi-level firms examined made false or misleading claims about their products in their promotional materials handed out by distributors.

⊘ Products such as vitamins that claimed nutritional value were "invariably overpriced." Across the board, direct marketing company supplements "generally cost much more than similar products" that are purchased through retail outlets.

⊘ Direct marketing distributors, in order to compete with retail outlets, must convince their prospective customers "that their products are superior, even though [in most cases] they are not."

⊘ Most of the direct marketing companies selling supplements "get their raw ingredients from the same bulk wholesalers and merely repackage them into brand-name products."

This last point is worth some elaboration. Much of what these companies promote as their "unique" and "special" vitamin/mineral formulated products are simply generics that come from the same small group of five private label manufacturers in the United States that provide the bulk of materials: Arnet Pharmaceuticals Corp., in Davie, Florida; Botanical Laboratories, Inc., in Ferndale, Washington; Contract Pharmacal Corp., in Hauppauge, New York; Leiner Health Products, Inc., in Carson, California; and Perrigo Company, in Allegan, Michigan.

Because nearly all direct marketing companies and major retail distributors get their supplement materials from the same basic suppliers, that means most direct marketed products are simply no better—or worse—in quality than the standard supplement company products.

In fairness to people involved with direct marketing programs, it should be pointed out that many people who are selling supplements and giving nutritional advice are not qualified to do so, and that includes nearly all physicians. Few medical schools even offer comprehensive courses on nutrition. Many non-medical people with a passion for vegan nutrition—some of whom may distribute plant- and food-based direct marketed products—know far more about authentic nutrition than most doctors, many of whom also distribute private-label chemical supplements. Additionally, most Western-trained dieticians and nutritionists, until recently, have been schooled in the chemical paradigm, rather than the whole-food, naturally occurring paradigm, when it comes to supplements, specifically in the benefits of consuming isolated (chemical) nutrients—the foundational and flawed assumption upon which the entire vitamin industry was built beginning 100 years ago.

New Technologies and Claims of Superiority

Higher prices do not mean higher quality! An examination of numerous products and their ingredients, and the associated Websites of supplement manufacturers, presents consumers with the following picture.

Some advertise their supplements as being "all-natural," free of preservatives, colorings, and other artificial additives, but if you examine their ingredients closely you will still find that the nutrients are synthetic and not from naturally occurring sources at all. Others say their nutrients are "modeled after nature," which is a dead giveaway that these are synthetics. Just duplicating in a laboratory the molecular structure of a nutrient does not mean that the synthetic will behave like a molecule from nature once it is inside the human body.

Organic is sometimes placed on labels even when the product's ingredients are a mix of organic and synthetic. Still others claim "high potency" supplements provide us with an important extra dose of a particular chemical that, based on our experience, is harmful in the first place. And they are charging more for it.

Finally, consider the safety implications of what is being done to supplements in the name of "product innovation" and "special features." In an attempt to prompt the human body to more readily absorb a greater percentage of nutrients from supplements, some companies using synthetic ingredients in their supplements are experimenting with the addition of nano-sized particles in both vitamins and inorganic minerals to facilitate absorption into cells.

Nanotechnology is being introduced at every level of the world economy, from plastics and textiles to sunblocks and cosmetics. So it was inevitable that nano-particles would turn up in supplements. Nano-particles can be as small as 100,000th the thickness of a sheet of paper, and this tiny size enables chemicals to enter the bloodstream and penetrate cells and body organs in a way never before possible with conventional chemicals.

But does shrinking the particles of synthetics down to this tiny size create safety problems we should be concerned about? "The chemicals industry has blithely assumed that if large grains are safe, smaller ones will be too," concluded *Nature*, the science journal, in a 2006 article titled "Nanoparticles in Sun Creams Can Stress Brain Cells." "But that assumption is coming under increasing scrutiny and is not necessarily always valid."

Emerging health concerns associated with nano-particles were well summarized in a November 22, 2007, article titled "A little risky business" in Britain's *The Economist* magazine: "Research on animals suggests that nano-particles can evade some of the body's natural defence systems and accumulate in the brain, cells, blood and nerves. Studies show there is the potential for such materials to reach the lung and cause inflammation...to other organs; to have surprising biological toxicity...."

You will need to read product labels even more carefully than ever before to detect the presence of nano-particles, if they are listed on labels at all. One giveaway will be if you see the terms *micro-fine* or *ultra-fine* associated with the ingredients listed.

CHAPTER 9

BEWARE OF THE "FOOD SOURCE" VITAMIN SCAM

A certain type of vitamin product manufactured by several companies claims to be from a "food source," but it's really a synthetic that has been cleverly disguised. Though it may look natural and have natural-appearing label claims, it's not natural at all.

These synthetic products are portrayed as being from "whole foods" or "food source," or something similar. They almost never claim that their vitamin potencies are "naturally occurring," as this would be a lie, but instead they use a label claim of "food source" or "whole food" vitamin potencies.

How can they make false statements on the label if the product contains synthetics? Because of a loophole in label claim law. *Here is how they do it:* The vitamin product is made with a base of algae or yeast that comes from a manufacturer that has "grown" the algae, yeast, or other bacterial-based material by adding synthetic vitamins to this base to create a certain "multiple" vitamin profile. The original bacterial base material (algae, yeast, or other bacterial or other materials) is spiked in large reactors or tanks with synthetic vitamins, creating a fermentation environment where the bacteriums (the yeast, algae, or other material) "grows," feeds on, or is forced to absorb the synthetic vitamins fed to this fermentation or other mixture. After the mixture is saturated with the spiked synthetic vitamins, the mixture is dried into a powder and shipped out to the vitamin manufacturers who use this base material for their "whole food" or "food source" vitamin products.

The vitamin company that uses this finished "whole food" vitamin material spiked with synthetics then creates a vitamin formula tablet or capsule using this base material that has a specific, lower, potency vitamin profile. When they put this material into their finished multiple-vitamin formulas, they can make a legal label claim saying that the spiked base material vitamin potencies are "natural" and from "whole food." The whole food they are referring to on the label is the base of algae, yeast, or other bacterium or food medium that was spiked with *synthetic* vitamins. This is legal because the synthetic vitamins were added to the base claimed as a "whole food" and not added directly to the finished product, and so they do not have to tell you that you are getting synthetic vitamin potencies *indirectly* from the base they use, *but you are getting the synthetic vitamins indirectly.*

This practice of "sneaking in" synthetic vitamins indirectly into your food supplements and labeling them as "natural" and from "whole food" or "food source" is a very deceptive practice designed to mislead consumers.

Why do they do this? Producers of synthetic vitamin materials have dominated the market for more than 70 years, and they don't want to lose market share by allowing you to recognize that their materials are synthetic, toxic chemical compounds.

The companies that use these "spiked" synthetic vitamin bases in their products can be identified by reading their labels. If the label of the suspect product has lower-than-usual vitamin potencies and mentions that these potencies are "from food source" or "from whole food" or something similar, but doesn't say "from naturally occurring food extracts" and names the actual food, then you have a right to suspect that the product may be spiked with synthetic vitamins. Most of the companies offering these spiked products and misleading labels are found within the "high-end" sections of natural food stores and other higher-end retailers, which means they charge a lot more for these products than you would pay for a regular synthetic vitamin.

If you want really, truly natural vitamins, then find those vitamin products that state on their label that their vitamin or mineral or nutrient potencies come from "Naturally Occurring Food Sources" *and* mention on their label which exact foods those sources are. Also, any vitamin products that carry the NOS (Naturally Occurring Standard) logo are safe and guaranteed to have vitamin potencies that only come from real, whole foods.

About 30 years ago a company called Golden Epoch made real, NOS vitamin and mineral supplements and found a niche market of people who wanted to get away from synthetic vitamin products. Golden Epoch did pretty well, even back then, but something happened. After about five years certain companies emerged using the spiked mediums containing synthetic vitamins as the base for their products, and these companies competed with Golden Epoch, claiming they had the same thing or better at the same or better price. It normally costs more to make a real NOS vitamin than it does to use the cheaper spiked material and make a misleading label claim, so these dishonest companies drove Golden Epoch out of business.

Was it a conspiracy or just ignorance and greed? Maybe the question doesn't matter anymore, because now you, the consumer, knows the truth about vitamins so you can see past all the myths. The final decision about whether synthetic vitamins or natural vitamins will prevail in our society belongs to the enlightened consumer. First the consumer has to know the truth, and only then can the right choice, the healthier choice, be made. We invite you to support the cause!

Are You Really Getting What You Pay For?

Yes, it is a myth that direct marketing products are necessarily superior to what you find in retail stores and doctor's offices, but it is also a myth that what you get in most retail stores and doctors' offices is superior to products marketed directly to you. In terms of superiority, there is only one question: Is it NOS or not NOS? Unless the answer is NOS, you are getting nothing of what you think you are paying for. Let's take a closer look at the costs to you, the consumer.

Because direct marketing distributors make money by purchasing supplements wholesale from the parent company and reselling them at a profit, and by receiving commissions from sponsoring others who resell at a profit, the markup on the product price above and beyond the cost of producing the product can be substantial. These network costs equal—and often exceed—retail store costs, which must factor in wholesalers, store employees, marketing, advertising, and so on, to the prices they charge.

An industry insider, who has worked with both direct marketing companies and retail stores in selling supplements, put the economics of production costs into focus this way. Synthetic vitamin C, for example, is relatively cheap to produce in a laboratory compared to naturally occurring vitamin C. You can picture the difference this way: Chemists in a lab isolate and extract the "active ingredient" of vitamin C, which they say is ascorbic acid, then they duplicate it cheaply using a synthetic chemical process on a production line. By contrast, naturally occurring vitamin C is extracted from an actual plant or fruit, which requires labor-intensive harvesting. Then it undergoes processing that condenses the essence of that plant or fruit—along with all of its important nutrient cofactors—into a dense nutrient pill, powder, or liquid form.

So the ultimate cost of growing and harvesting the plant, fruit, or herb source, the cost of shipping it for processing, the cost of extraction, and the cost of actual processing all combined together results in a higher price than most synthetics. Given that economic reality, if you see synthetics that are the same price or higher than the same type of supplements taken from a natural source, your consumer alarm bells should start ringing! Production of synthetic vitamin C costs 80- to 90-percent less per unit of value (potency claimed) than whole-food naturally occurring vitamin C, which is the main reason why synthetics bought from bulk suppliers are so attractive to most supplement manufacturers, including those in the direct marketing field.

If a manufacturer buys a finished vitamin product from a bulk manufacturer for, let's say, $3, after production, marketing, and distribution costs (which vary based on the type of distribution—retail versus direct marketing), the price will be anywhere from $12 to $15 (wholesale). The general retail markup is typically 100 percent over wholesale, so a consumer will pay around $30 retail for a product that actually costs less than $8 to manufacture. Consumers can count on a minimum retail price/cost ratio of 10 to 1, for a chemical product that may also be "costing" you your health.

In contrast, the base cost of a purely whole-food vitamin supplement that is organic and NOS certified is approximately two to three times the base price of the synthetic vitamin product from a bulk manufacturer. Retail prices are understandably higher for NOS products as compared to their synthetic counterparts—however, not *much* higher. Keep in mind also that in many cases lower dosages of NOS supplements can be used to achieve the desired results, simply because the supplements can be fully utilized by the body, which offsets their higher retail expense. One additional point on the pricing of NOS supplements: Because NOS supplements cost more to produce, their value is not yet fully recognized by consumers. As such, the retail markup over wholesale on some NOS supplements can be as low as 50 percent to remain "competitive," even though the products offered by the "competition" are synthetic and of far lesser quality and value.

As we noted earlier, the cost of some products distributed through direct marketing channels can be higher because of the commission and incentive programs that are in place to drive the building of downline networks, and because of their own beliefs of superior product quality. The industry publication *Nutraceuticals World* featured an article by Rebecca Madley in a July 2001 issue in which numerous direct marketing company executives were quoted as giving various justifications for their supplement prices being higher than those in retail stores. "In terms of our products, you can't find them anywhere else, so we have a unique proposition," said one executive.

A president of one of the larger direct marketing firms said that direct marketing is like a doctor who makes house calls: "A doctor who makes house calls would probably charge you more than a doctor who makes you come to his office, e.g. our approach to one-on-one marketing versus retail. We pay our people more."

One direct marketing company even makes this claim on its Website about why it has higher prices: "Products that are more expensive usually have greater features and benefits over competitive products."

But when it comes to synthetic nutrients taken from the same bulk suppliers, their attempts to compete about quality are mostly an illusion. Supplement sellers that rely upon synthetic ingredients are competing with each other based more on marketing strategies and branding claims than on true product quality differences.

To illustrate this point, a February 2008 Associated Press investigation revealed how a direct marketing company marketed a nutrient drink at nearly $40 a bottle, calling it an antioxidant immunity booster. But when the product was tested in a lab at Oregon State University's Linus Pauling Institute, it was found to have antioxidant strength no greater than a comparable-sized product sold for just $3 or less at retail stores. Consumers were paying 10 times the price they would for comparable products because they believed the stories of health benefits being told as part of the company's marketing strategy. As Anthony Almada, president and chief executive of GENr8 Inc., a dietary supplement company, admitted to the Associated Press: "The industry is built on storytelling, and because they do it one-on-one, without advertising, they don't incur the wrath of the FDA."

Although you might be alarmed to learn this, vitamin supplement manufacturers across the board, and regardless of distribution methods, are freeing themselves from liability by using the simple phrase "this statement has not been evaluated by the FDA." In these cases, if the supplement does not carry the NOS certification, we advise you to inquire further about the vitamin source.

The stark reality of today is that few sources of supplements, be they standard supplement distributors, from doctors, or from direct marketing companies, offer naturally occurring vitamins and minerals that have been proven to be completely free of all synthetic ingredients, including colorings and other additives. Yet they are charging consumers as if they were. Although we could debate the issue of high markups in the vitamin-supplement industry, it is difficult to debate—in the case of chemical supplements—that you are getting far less than what you believed you were paying for, and perhaps far more than you bargained for.

We encourage all companies, no matter what marketing system they use, to abandon synthetics, which are overpriced and with unproven or over-valued health benefits. We urge them to instead develop only plant-based non-synthetic products as a service to the cause of public health.

CHAPTER 10

RECOMMENDED DAILY ALLOWANCES SPREAD CONFUSION

Our culture's entire structure of nutritional standards, from the Recommended Daily Allowance (RDA) model for our nutrient intake to a range of other dietary guidelines established by governments and research institutes, have mostly been built on synthetic chemicals that try to imitate natural foods.

If this system was the Great Pyramid of Egypt, it would be a pile of rubble by now because the base would be imitation stone made from shifting sand. It is a system erected almost entirely on a hierarchy of faulty premises and assumptions about the relative equivalence of synthetic and natural nutrients.

RDAs were established to be dosage guidelines for everyone who consumes vitamins and minerals, with the intention being to create a minimal level of public health. It was a standard designed to prevent diseases caused by deficiencies, a purpose for which it has far outlived its usefulness. The very idea that RDAs can be applied equally to everyone ignores how widely our individual nutrient needs vary, especially based on our lifestyle choices. Those who consume meat, for instance, will carry a body burden of synthetic chemicals and resulting nutrient deficiencies that do not plague people who are vegans or vegetarians.

During World War II the Recommended Daily Allowance (RDA) model for nutrients, including vitamins, was established by the National Academy of Sciences as a general guideline for feeding American soldiers. This model went through several changes and revisions throughout the years, until in 1997 the USDA replaced the term *RDA* with *RDI* (Reference Daily Intake). This U.S. standard is now employed worldwide.

Nutrition expert T. Colin Campbell, a professor of nutritional biochemistry at Cornell University and author of *The China Study*, served on the most recent National Academy of Sciences committee on food labeling, which was responsible for redesigning the RDA information. He has since pointed out, in an article titled "RDAs: Time to Peel Back the Labels" on NutritionAdvocate.com, how "it's a recommended allowance; it's not a *minimum* requirement...in other words, to play it safe, the RDA represents a substantially higher intake than what you need."

Here is a key problem with the RDA approach that Campbell identifies. These RDAs are biased toward supporting diets that are high in fat, high in animal protein, and low in fiber—the same diet that causes us so many health problems. Beta-carotene, which comes mostly from plants, does not even have an RDA, nor does dietary fiber, another plant-based nutrient.

"When it comes time to hand out RDAs," observes Campbell, "plant-based nutrients are either not assigned one or are given an RDA biased toward the low side. By contrast, RDAs for animal-based nutrients are characteristically biased upwards." Professor Campbell goes on to declare that RDAs "have mostly been an albatross around the neck of sound nutrition education."

There are other drawbacks regarding these nutritional standards. The board that established them admits that scientific knowledge of nutritional requirements is far from complete, and, as a result, the requirements for many nutrients have not been established. It also admits that in all likelihood other nutrients will be found to be essential in years to come.

We must also keep in mind that the studies used to determine the level of a nutrient sufficient to prevent a nutritional deficiency were typically conducted for six to nine months—less than 1 percent of the average human life span. So a case can be made that nutritional standards were extrapolated from incomplete data.

Nutritional studies with animals have shown that the amounts of some nutrients sufficient to provide health and aid in the prevention of a deficiency disease for short periods may be totally inadequate to maintain health throughout an entire lifespan. The RDAs are based on scientific research in both humans and animals and are supposedly set at levels to accommodate 98 percent of all healthy persons. There is a built-in cushion: theoretically, if you get 67 percent of the RDA from a nutrient, you are getting acceptable amounts.

People are increasingly confused about what to eat, how to eat, and when to eat. A 1996 USDA survey verified this when 40 percent of respondents agreed strongly with the statement that "there are so many recommendations about healthy ways to eat, it's hard to know what to believe."

Part of the growing dietary confusion has to do with a concept called the Daily Value (DV). Introduced by the USDA in the 1990s, the DV is a dietary reference that is supposed to guide people to make healthy eating choices. Daily Values are made up of both DRVs—Daily Reference Value (which keeps track of proteins, carbohydrates, fats, cholesterol, and so on) and RDIs—Recommended Daily Intake (which was designed for essential vitamins and minerals).

The DV informs consumers how many nutrients they are getting from a particular food item. For example, if the DV label on a can of peas states that it represents "10 percent of the DV for fat," consumers can keep track of that number and know throughout the day how much fat they are ingesting. It is supposed to estimate the amount of a nutrient needed by an average healthy person to avoid showing signs of deficiency. The recommendations have built-in safety margins, so in many cases the DV far exceeds the minimum amount of a nutrient. Most children and adults can thrive on 50 percent of some of the recommendations.

The minimum level of vitamin C needed to prevent scurvy, for example, is around 10 milligrams per day for the average person. In the government suggestions, the DV is set at 60 milligrams to allow for individuals who may require more vitamin C, but Professor Campbell suggests that levels closer to 200 to 300 milligrams a day would be more beneficial for overall maximum health.

The DV specifies the minimum of a nutrient needed to stay healthy. This concept is not to be confused with the amount of nutrients the body actually uses or needs, because we typically absorb much less of a nutrient than is actually found in the food.

The research and studies that have been conducted as related to vitamins, minerals, and certain nutrients for RDAs and other standards were done using mainly synthetic compound quantities. So what, then, is the true value of such standards as the RDAs, DVs, RDIs, and other acronym standards, based upon synthetic quantities?

One More Myth Busted

Because these recommendations are based upon research using synthetics, then the standards that follow from these recommendations neither relate nor apply to natural food-derived vitamins, minerals, and other nutrients.

In the case of carbohydrates, fats, proteins, and other non-vitamin or nutrient quantities, these standards may hold up. But to develop a standard such as an RDA for a real, naturally occurring vitamin, it would be necessary to use an extract of a full-spectrum source of that vitamin, not a synthetic from some laboratory, as the standard-setting test material.

It is obvious that the people who set up these standards did not understand or appreciate the difference, as outlined in this book, between synthetic chemical supplements and whole-food supplements. Did they begin with the premise that synthetic chemicals, similar to synthetic vitamins, are the same as *real* vitamins and nutrients? It seems they did, which was their original mistake.

This is why it is confusing to use RDAs, DVs, or RDIs to determine our daily intake of natural vitamins and nutrients. We suggest that you focus instead on consuming a balanced whole-food diet with proper whole-food based supplementation.

It is not possible for the committees that calculate the DVs to present optimal values for every person and every situation. The DV numbers are only based upon the amount a person needs to keep from getting sick or seriously ill, plus a margin of error. Daily allowances were initially created for young and active military males, meaning that they are almost certainly less appropriate for the very young, the elderly, and women.

DVs are particularly outdated when it comes to the recommended level of antioxidant nutrients such as vitamin C, vitamin E, and beta carotene. Some nutritionists believe the DVs for these health-promoting nutrients should be at least two to five times their current values, but that may be too high for some individuals, especially when a person is consuming large amounts of toxic synthetic vitamins as supplements and again through food fortification.

Christine Lewis, PhD, a registered dietician and director of the division of technical evaluation in the FDA's Office of Food Labeling, has said, "The DV term is the one we expect consumers and professionals to use. They're not recommended intakes. They are really just reference points to help people get some kind of perspective on what their overall daily dietary needs should be."

Of course, if the DV is related to a synthetic vitamin value rather than a real and complete vitamin derived from food, it obviously falls short of being much use to anyone.

The move to Daily Values is due in part to the Nutrition Labeling and Education Act of 1990. The law requires nutrition label information to be conveyed in a way that enables the public to observe and comprehend the information readily and to understand its relative significance in the context of a total daily diet. FDA-regulated products such as vitamins were required to begin using the Daily Values as the basis for declaring nutrient content on labels on May 8, 1994.

Review of Nutrient Standard Terms

1. DVs (Daily Values): a new dietary reference term that will appear on the food label. It is made up of two sets of references: DRVs and RDIs.

2. DRVs (Daily Reference Values): a set of dietary references that applies to fat, saturated fat, cholesterol, carbohydrate, protein, fiber, sodium, and potassium.

3. RDIs (Reference Daily Intakes): a set of dietary references based on the Recommended Dietary Allowances for essential vitamins and minerals, and, in selected groups, protein. The name "RDI" replaces the term *U.S. RDA*. (The difference between RDI and RDA is that RDI is based upon a number of calories of food per day; for example: "2,000-calorie diet for adults." And RDA does not generally make a calorie-per-day distinction).

4. RDAs (Recommended Dietary Allowances): a set of estimated nutrient allowances established by the National Academy of Sciences that is updated periodically to reflect current scientific knowledge.

Refusing to Play the Synthetics Game

RDAs, DVs, and RDIs are all part of the synthetic-vitamin milligram game. Because there is no standard based upon non-synthetic, naturally occurring vitamins, real organic minerals, or other nutrient values, we have founded a nonprofit organization that will pioneer these new standards in the coming years.

Having no natural nutrient standards can be a big problem for those of us who want to take a daily amount of a real, naturally occurring multiple-vitamin and mineral supplements. How do we know how much to take? And what can we do about it?

First, we have to give our support to the few companies that make whole, naturally occurring full-spectrum food supplements. Make sure they put the vitamin values/potencies on their labels, too, as this important information seems scarce these days. (See Appendix C for sources.)

The question is: If a synthetic vitamin RDI for synthetic vitamin C (ascorbic acid) is 60 mgs per day, then how much of a truly naturally occurring vitamin C product supplement should we take?

A common sense answer is that you probably do not need a synthetic's quantity as a guide because the nutrient is real, naturally occurring, and therefore more effective. With this reasoning you may decide that only half as much or less of a naturally occurring vitamin C—say, 15 to 30 mgs instead of 60 mgs of synthetic C—will accomplish the same results or better. Fifteen milligrams might even be better, if the source of those milligrams is a whole, naturally occurring source.

The real problem is that there is no simple answer. Everyone's daily dose of vitamins and nutrients is unique, depending on age, gender, health, dietary habits, and stress levels. We believe you can use fewer milligrams of a naturally occurring food source of a vitamin or nutrient and receive better results than from the same dosage of a synthetic vitamin or nutrient, and do so without the harmful side effects that can include a weakened immune system.

Until we have our own Naturally Occurring Standard (NOS), which will be created out of years of clinical research, we have to live with the current RDAs. So treat them simply as guidelines, not as appropriate or final answers to our real needs.

So...how do we determine our daily intake of necessary nutrients?

For the time being, the answer is to take some whole-food supplementation daily, even if it does not equal or exceed current synthetic standards. The point is that you need a vital potency, not a synthetic or non-organic one. Real potency, even when lower than a higher-potency synthetic, will provide the building blocks that allow every organ to strengthen and function better.

Today even well-meaning health professionals have no clue that synthetic vitamins are harmful and ineffective, because they have trusted standards based on synthetic vitamins and nutrients as established by the National Research Council. So we have a lot of educational work to do.

You can help in this effort by purchasing only whole nutrients and organic whole foods. We also need to demand that governments and their health departments change the standards and transform daily nutrient requirements to include Natural Daily Allowances (NDAs) that reflect the Naturally Occurring Standard (NOS) approach to scientific accuracy and the advancement of optimal public health.

CHAPTER 11

LEGAL STRUCTURES TO PROTECT THE NATURAL STANDARD

Our freedom to choose the supplements we want and need for good health has come under an unprecedented challenge from an alliance between government agencies and the global pharmaceutical industry.

By distorting the distinctions between synthetic and naturally occurring products and substances, these agencies and economic interests are trying to ensure our reliance on the synthetics belief system through tighter regulatory restraints. Such restraints, done in the name of protecting public health, end up most directly benefiting the huge corporations that manipulate government decision-making.

No one should be surprised that this challenge to our nutritional freedom has materialized at a time when greater numbers of people are using naturally occurring products.

Numerous books and exposés have appeared throughout the years showing how the U.S. Food and Drug Administration, charged with regulating foods, drugs, and supplements, has been unduly influenced by the global food processing and pharmaceutical industries. The same is also becoming true of the European Union, which has undertaken a global assault on natural healthcare, starting with nutrients.

That all too familiar statement, "We have the best government that money can buy," has often been applied to the FDA, its officials, and their decisions. The agency does receive much of its funding from the industries it is supposed to regulate, and the revolving door, in which FDA officials take jobs with corporations they previously oversaw as regulators, ensures that the FDA is responsive to industry wishes. Representatives of this agency have actually confessed that the large pharmaceutical industries are their true clients, rather than we consumers, and this candor reinforces the perception that misplaced priorities dominate their agenda.

Throughout the years the FDA has made a few good decisions, but far too many bad ones regarding food supplements and nutraceuticals. Too often we see the restriction or removal of a natural product once it competes effectively with highly funded and heavily lobbied pharmaceutical products. Sometimes, however, the FDA's actions are fully justified, as with the excellent ruling restricting ephedrine alkaloids in food supplements.

Ephedrine alkaloids are chemical compounds commonly found in the herb ephedra, a popular weight-loss-product ingredient. The FDA ruling, as found in the Federal Register, concluded in February 11, 2004: "dietary supplements containing ephedrine alkaloids (ephedra)...present an unreasonable risk of illness or injury."

The chief problem with ephedrine alkaloids as found in the ephedra herb is abuse. Some food-supplement companies were making weight-loss products with extremely high levels of ephedrine alkaloids. High concentrations of ephedrine, which do not occur in the raw, natural ephedra herb, act like a drug in the human body, resembling the effects of amphetamines.

Large pharmaceutical companies support the idea of regulating all vitamins as drugs, which would give them an even bigger competitive advantage in the marketplace. This idea is already a reality in Germany, where the law now requires anyone who wants high doses of vitamins to obtain a prescription from a licensed medical doctor.

Throughout Europe, ever-increasing restrictions are being placed on the promotion of natural, whole-food supplements and herbs. This attempt to place more control in the hands of government agencies for the sale and distribution of supplements is spreading to North America.

The Threat Posed by Codex Standards

Your freedom to use vitamins at dosage levels unique to your biochemistry and particular to your health needs may be in serious jeopardy. Below the radar scan of mainstream media attention, an international organization has been formulating hundreds of standards and rules that will affect how the entire world regulates the sale of food, and vitamins and minerals, including at what dosage levels they can be sold without a prescription from a physician.

Known as Codex Alimentarius, which is Latin for "food code," it was established by the United Nations to create international rules governing all aspects of the trade in food and nutrition products, from production to distribution. These standards affect vitamins and minerals irrespective of whether they are derived from synthetic or natural sources. Ostensibly, the first and primary purpose of these international rules, as stated in Codex Statute, Article 1(a) is: "protecting the health of the consumers and ensuring fair practices in the food trade."

Although this may sound all well and good, there is a problem: As the old saying goes, "the devil is in the details." Codex standards are scheduled for global implementation by December 31, 2009, and are based on Napoleonic Code principles rather than the common law principles used throughout the modern world. Under the Napoleonic Code, anything not explicitly permitted by written law is therefore illegal. By contrast, common law takes the opposite approach—anything not explicitly *banned* in written law is automatically permitted.

Ratified by the Codex Commission on July 4, 2005, the rules on vitamins and minerals that the governments of the world are being pressured to adopt as their domestic law include the following "devils in the details" that are relevant to you and this book:

⊘ Supplements, the rules stipulate, "should contain vitamins/provitamins and minerals whose nutritional value for human beings has been proven by scientific data and whose status as vitamins and minerals is recognized by FAO (Food and Agriculture Organization) and WHO (World Health Organization)." These are both United Nations groups.

⊘ The sources of vitamins and minerals "may be either natural or synthetic and their selection should be based on considerations such as safety and bioavailability. In addition, purity criteria should take into account FAO/WHO standards."

⊘ "The minimum level of each vitamin and/or mineral contained in a vitamin and mineral food supplement per daily portion of consumption as suggested by the manufacturer, should be 15 percent of the recommended daily intake as determined by FAO/WHO."

⊘ Maximum amounts of vitamins and minerals in supplements "shall take the following criteria into account: upper safe levels of vitamins and minerals established by scientific risk assessment based on generally accepted scientific data."

Any vitamin and mineral supplement that meets the guidelines (among many others) detailed here, as set by the Codex Commission, can be imported into any nation that has adopted as its domestic law a Model International Dietary Supplement Act, written by the Codex Commission. If the nations that don't adopt these Codex rules and the model act attempt to interfere in the international trade of supplements based on their own domestic laws, they will face international trade sanctions by the World Trade Organization. In other words, nations must "harmonize" their own laws with Codex in order to continue participating in the world food and supplements economy.

Three dozen different Codex committees have been formulating the various standards and rules throughout the past decade, but the one that concerns us most, for the purposes of this book, is the Committee on Nutrition on Foods for Special Dietary Uses. That committee, which oversees supplements, has been headed by a German physician, Rolf Grossklaus, who has played an extremely important role in shaping the rules pertaining to permissible dosage levels in supplements. Dr. Grossklaus was the coauthor of a report done by the German Risk Assessment Institute in 2005, of which he is chairman of the board, which performed a toxicology analysis of supplements and then prepared maximum allowable dosage levels. This report has become the Codex Commission model for international dosage standards, thanks largely to Dr. Grossklaus being in charge of the Codex committee, with jurisdiction over supplements.

The exceptionally low allowable potencies that resulted from this exercise would effectively end our freedom to use therapeutic doses of vitamins on our own initiative. Any dosage levels above the maximum would either be banned outright, or regulated by the necessity to obtain doctor's prescriptions for their use. For instance, here are a few of the stark contrasts between the "recommended" levels currently set by the U.S. Food and Nutrition Board, versus the "mandatory" maximum levels set by German/Codex standards:

⊘ Vitamin C: 2,000 mg in the U.S.; 225 mg under Codex.

⊘ Vitamin E: 1,000 mg in the U.S.; 15 mg under Codex.

⊘ Vitamin B6: 100 mg in the U.S.; 5.4 mg under Codex.

What becomes clear from reading the entire list in which unnecessarily low dosage ceilings are set is that Dr. Grossklaus and the Codex Commission view the nutrients in supplements—even when they are derived from natural food sources—to be little more than toxins in need of regulation because they pose hazards to health. This is an approach that uses risk-assessment models already in place for pharmaceutical drugs and other synthetic chemical toxins.

As you may already know based on your own experience with supplements and from reading this book, this Codex point of view is grossly in error both in its science methodology and in its attitude toward natural products. To regulate food-based nutritional supplements as if they were toxins, as these rules would do, not only restricts our freedom to choose natural approaches to health but represents a rejection of the entire history of human experience with nature and its life-affirming nutrients.

These Codex proposals have been in force in Norway and Germany since 2005, when the entire health-food industry in those countries was undermined by large, multi-national drug companies using Codex as a pretext for implementing restrictions of access to natural nutrients.

In these countries, vitamin C above 200 mg, vitamin E above 45 IU and vitamin B1 above 2.4 mg—and many others—are now available only by prescription. As you can imagine, many natural-foods enthusiasts there are outraged, and rightfully so.

Norwegian pharmaceutical giant Shering-Plough now controls echinacea tincture. It is sold in Norway as an over-the-counter drug at grossly inflated prices. The same is true of ginkgo biloba and many other herbs, because only one government-controlled pharmacy has the right to import supplements as medicines to sell to pharmacies, natural food stores, and convenience stores.

The major European pharmaceutical companies and medical associations support the Codex agenda of restricting vitamin supplements in Europe—and soon in the United States—not because it is good for the consumer, but because it makes good business sense. Maximizing profits, not protecting health freedoms, motivates these institutions to manipulate government bureaucrats and public officials until everyone is "harmonized" with the same agenda.

What are the odds of the U.S. Food and Drug Administration embracing these draconian Codex standards and rules? In a notice published in the Federal Register in October 1995, the FDA announced its intention to "harmonize its regulatory requirements" to reflect Codex standards and to abide by international trade agreements, particularly those implemented by the World Trade Organization. There has been no indication that the FDA will retreat from that position. Health freedom would be sacrificed to avoid the economic repercussions of failing to follow the Codex and WTO dictates.

This situation places the Codex standards on a collision course with a 1994 law passed by the U.S. Congress, the Dietary Supplement Health and Education Act, that effectively reaffirms supplement health freedom for American citizens by placing no upper limits on nutrient dosages. In America, more than 50 percent of the population takes a daily vitamin or food supplement. If the Codex legislation gets implemented here, the big pharmaceutical companies could corner the market on vitamins and remove any competition by the natural foods and nutraceutical industry.

Although we might agree with the concept of controlling synthetic vitamins—which, after all, are drugs—what we do find objectionable is the idea of an international committee dictating what food or food supplements we can and cannot take as part of our own personal healthcare choices.

The Alliance for Natural Health (ANH) in Surrey, United Kingdom, a nonprofit organization and consumer advocate group, has been fighting against these moves to restrict consumers' rights to free access to vitamins, food supplements, and alternative nutritional and medical therapies. The alliance has been able to report at least one major victory with a lawsuit against the European Courts of Justice (ECJ) to prevent future Codex restrictions of naturally occurring vitamin supplements in world markets. The alliance secured a ruling that vitamins and minerals found in the human diet were *not* a threat to public health and do not need to undergo constant safety evaluations. (For more information go to *www.alliance-natural-health.org*.)

The alliance's worldwide activities have resulted in substantial victories for those who cherish the freedom to choose their own diet and food supplements without interference, but much more work needs to be done, as evidenced by the threat posed by unrealistically low maximum dosage levels for supplements.

Eternal vigilance is the price of freedom, most especially of our health freedom. Natural nutrients are our rightful gift from nature. To defend that right and our access to nature's bounty, we must continually be aware that economic forces are at work advancing coercive agendas. We must speak out in every possible way, or our silence will be interpreted as consent.

AFTERWORD

A NEW STANDARD FOR YOUR LIFE

Now that you have absorbed the information in this book, what will you do with this knowledge? How will you apply it to your life? Start the inquiry by asking yourself the following questions:

- ⊘ Does your commitment to health—for yourself and for those you care about—now extend to studying all product labels to identify those containing synthetic ingredients?

- ⊘ Will you refuse to overpay and waste your money on synthetic vitamins now that you know your body cannot readily absorb them?

- ⊘ Are you now prepared to seek naturally occurring sources for the nutrients you know your body needs for immunity and good health?

- ⊘ Do you feel willing to tell others that we need to defend our right to choose non-synthetic nutrients and food products?

If your answer to any of these questions was in the affirmative, you are probably a good candidate for spreading the word about the importance of establishing a naturally occurring standard for vitamins, minerals, and foods in general. This standard will be a concise and clear beacon for those who want to make a statement on behalf of their own health and the public health.

We need naturally occurring vitamin supplements to be more widely accepted and available in the marketplace. But until the public can clearly distinguish between natural and synthetic, our choices and our health will be at the mercy of those economic institutions that profit from sowing confusion.

NOS will be a label affixed to nutritional supplements and whole botanical products that come directly from the plants of nature and contain no synthetic ingredients of any kind. If you do not see the NOS designation on a product label, you will be able to assume that it contains synthetic chemicals. The NOS will also provide a way to certify the potencies of natural ingredients placed in vitamins and fortified foods.

A nonprofit organization has been formed, the Naturally Occurring Standards Group (NOSG), to promote the NOS label and guidelines for foods, vitamins, and medicines. This group will develop protocols and applications for NOS certification of products and will issue an NOS certification sticker for manufacturers that meets rigorous NOS criteria.

Our campaign goals are to implement NOS certification procedures and labels that are genuinely organic, while simultaneously educating consumers about the reality of how more than 90 percent of vitamins and supplements now being sold as "natural" or "food-based" are actually spiked with synthetic chemicals. That is a worldwide scandal and it needs to be exposed, which is why we urge you to tell your friends and associates about this book and about the NOS campaign.

We all need complete and accurate information about the contents of the products we purchase. You as a consumer deserve to be told the truth, and you deserve to have a range of options to be exercised by your judgment alone. Your nutritional freedom should not be subject to the arbitrary whims of regulatory bureaucrats, or to manipulation by drug makers, who are all in service to a synthetics belief system that ignores the wisdom of nature.

We can help to ensure the existence of a naturally occurring option for generations to come if we adopt the NOS as a code of business ethics for society and as a lifestyle choice for ourselves. The future really is in your hands.

(For more information about NOS and how you can get involved, go to *www.nosg.org*.)

APPENDIX A

NATURAL SOURCES OF VITAMINS, AND VITAMIN DEFICIENCY SYMPTOMS

At the Hippocrates Health Institute, where I am codirector, we conducted a two-year study of the health benefits of whole-food based supplementation. We separated 283 of our guests into two similarly sized groups based upon the relative strength or weakness of their immune system cells as measured in blood tests. These two broadly defined groups consisted of those who were "healthy" and those who were "unhealthy."

The components of each person's physiology that we considered included white blood cells (leukocytes), T-cells, H-cells, and such "differentials" as eosinophils, neutrifils, basophils, and lymphocytes. Those who displayed moderate or abundant immune strength were placed into the "healthy" group. In the "unhealthy" group were those who had moderately weak blood-test results and those who displayed minimal immune function.

We wanted to determine the importance of whole-food supplementation in the recovery and maintenance of the human body. Participants were assigned a whole food–based dietary supplement program designed to enhance immune function. Our study revealed an improvement of immune-system function in an average of 26 percent of the "unhealthy" participants as a result of naturally occurring supplements.

This degree of nutritional fulfilment can be the difference between life and death, but all too often people wait until they are seriously ill before attempting to improve their health by stopping self-destructive habits. For the seriously ill, someone who is near death, this process might be too gradual to generate complete recovery. It is here that bioactive, food-based nutrients are essential and life-altering.

Of the participants in the "healthy" group, approximately 7 percent realized improvement in immune function as a result of naturally occurring supplementation. This seemingly minimal percentage is nevertheless critical to those who expend a lot of energy in their daily activities—people with stressful responsibilities, including extensive travel; athletes; and pregnant women. The study also revealed that most of the participants in both groups needed to consume whole food–based supplements for about two years to restore consistent immune-cell balance and achieve complete functioning.

Here is a list of the sources, benefits, and potential risks of vitamins:

Vitamin A: Beta-Carotene; Retinol

Supplemental vitamin A should be consumed as beta-carotene, which is a precursor (manufacturer) of vitamin A.

Best sources: Sunflower green sprouts, green leafy vegetables, chia sprouts, sea vegetables, and cruciferous vegetables.

Major symptoms of vitamin A deficiency: Night blindness, dryness of various parts of the eye, and blindness.

Major symptoms of vitamin A toxicity: Liver damage, irritability, weakness, diminished menstrual bleeding, and psychiatric disorders.

Vitamin B1: Thiamin; Thiamine

Best sources: Wheatgrass, sprouted sweet potato, sprouted peas, sprouted corn, and raw sauerkraut.

Major symptoms of B1 deficiency: Beriberi, headaches, irritability, fatigue, lethargy, and neurological diseases.

Major symptoms of B1 toxicity: Allergic reactions.

Vitamin B2: Riboflavin (Formerly Cited as Vitamin G)

Best sources: Cabbage sprouts, kamut grass, raw corn, buckwheat-green sprouts, and corn sprouts.

Major symptoms of vitamin B2 deficiency: Soreness of the mouth and tongue, dermal and genital rashes, neuropathy, and anemia.

Major symptoms of vitamin B2 toxicity: Possible increase of tumor growth (and possible additional complications theretofore).

Vitamin B3: Niacin (Nicontinamide; Nicontinic Acid)

Best sources: Sprouted wheat, spelt, kamut grasses, sea kelp, and dulse.

Major symptoms of vitamin B3 deficiency: Circulatory and cardio-vascular disease.

Major symptoms of vitamin B3 toxicity: Burning, itching, headache, nausea, vomiting, duodenal ulcers, and liver failure.

Vitamin B5: Pantothenic Acid; Calcium Panthothenate

Best sources: Pecans, sprouted sesame seeds, avocado, organic apples, and apricot seeds.

Major symptoms of vitamin B5 deficiency: Respiratory infection, fatigue, cardiac irregularities, gastrointestinal complications, rashes, staggering, muscle cramps, and disorientation.

Major symptoms of vitamin B5 toxicity: Diarrhea and water retention.

Vitamin B6: Pyridoxine; Pyridoxal; Pyridoxamine

Best sources: Sprouted sweet potato, cabbage sprouts, wheatgrass, sprouted mango seed, and Brussels sprouts.

Major symptoms of vitamin B6 deficiency: Rashes, seizures, carpal tunnel syndrome, and anemia.

Major symptoms of vitamin B6 toxicity: Unsteadiness, muscle weakness, and systemic weakness.

Vitamin B12 (Considered a probiotic): Cobalamine; Cobalamin; Cyanocobalamine; Hydroxocobalamin

Best sources: Blue-green algae, raw tempeh, raw sauerkraut, organic green vegetable juice, and wheatgrass. **Supplement is needed daily.**

Major symptoms of vitamin B12 deficiency: Pernicious anemia, sometimes causing unpleasant internal electrical impulses permeating the lips, nose, and extremities; susceptibility to colds and other infections; bruising; and impaired blood clotting.

Major symptoms of vitamin B12 toxicity: Allergic reactions and rashes.

Vitamin C: Camu, Camu Berries, Manioc Root, Amla Berries

Best sources: Cauliflower, broccoli, black currants, sprouted papaya seed, and kiwi fruit.

Major symptoms of vitamin C deficiency: Scurvy and its symptoms (primarily spontaneous bleeding), edema and wounds that do not heal, cardiovascular disease, and cancer.

Major symptoms of vitamin C toxicity: Excessive urination and kidney stones.

Choline

Best sources: Onion sprouts, broccoli sprouts, cauliflower, grapes, and ripe tomatoes.

Major symptoms of choline deficiency: Impaired lung functioning.

Major symptoms of choline toxicity: Enlargement of the liver and the spleen, anemia, and increasing physical and mental degeneration.

Vitamin D

Best sources: Clover sprouts, arame seaweed, blue-green algae, sprouted pinto beans, and olives.

Major symptoms of vitamin D deficiency: Impaired vision; dermal impairment causing blotches, lack of tautness, and weakness of the skin, hair, and nails.

Major symptoms of vitamin D toxicity: Anemia, weakness, loss of appetite, vomiting, diarrhea, kidney failure, and death.

Vitamin E

Best sources: Sunflower green sprouts, sprouted almonds, sprouted filberts, sprouted pine nuts, and avocado.

Major symptoms of vitamin E deficiency: Anemia, weakness, and degeneration of the spinal cord and peripheral nerves.

Major symptoms of vitamin E toxicity: Nausea, flatulence, diarrhea, and allergic contact dermatitis.

Folate: Folic Acid

Best sources: Beet-root greens, broccoli sprouts, all lettuce, sprouted garbanzo beans, and sprouted black-eyed peas.

Major symptoms of folic acid deficiency: Miscarriage, complications of pregnancy, birth defects, neurological malfunction, and heart disease.

Major symptoms of folic acid toxicity: Renal toxicity causing kidney enlargement and possible kidney failure.

Vitamin H: Biotin

Best sources: Raw sesame tahini, sprouted almonds, walnuts, sprouted filberts, and hemp seeds.

Major symptoms of biotin deficiency: Disorientation, tremors, loss of memory, speech impairment; unsteady gait, and "restless legs."

Major symptoms of biotin toxicity: Cartilage erosion.

Vitamin K

Best sources: Sea kelp, broccoli sprouts, cabbage sprouts, alfalfa sprouts, and kale.

Major symptoms of vitamin K deficiency: Blood dilution.

Major symptoms of vitamin K toxicity: Blood clotting.

Appendix B

The Naturally Occurring Standard Abstract

Note to Readers: The following science abstract was prepared by the author for submission to research institutes and the supplements industry. It summarizes the case to be made for adopting a Naturally Occurring Standard for the industry and consumers, and it shows how this standard would work in practice as a certification and public education tool.

THE NATURALLY OCCURRING STANDARD
Brian Clement, NMD, PhD, and Scott Treadway, PhD
Hippocrates Health Institute, West Palm Beach, Florida

Abstract

The Naturally Occurring Standard (NOS) is being established for the purpose of identifying, certifying, labeling, and verifying the naturally occurring vitamins and nutrients in all food products, including bulk food materials, nutritional supplements, and fortified foods, and for the purpose of expressing a clear distinction between naturally occurring vitamins and nutrient-containing products and those that contain synthetic vitamins and nutrients. The current quantitative and qualitative standards for vitamins and other essential nutrients, such as those listed by RDAs, RDIs, and DVs, for understanding nutrient activity, label disclosure, and other nutrient details related to food supplements and fortified foods, are originally based upon synthetic quantities mostly developed upon animal research studies conducted more than 60 years ago.

There is no qualitative or quantitative standard currently available for understanding non-synthetic, naturally occurring vitamin and nutrient potencies for the purpose of labeling or publication as related to our fortified foods and dietary supplements. This situation is confusing in general not only for natural food supplement and food product developers, but also for consumers, who should be informed about the distinction that exists between naturally occurring vitamins and nutrients obtained only and directly from food, and botanical sources created by nature, as opposed to manmade synthetic vitamins and nutrients produced in laboratories. Therefore, a new standard, the NOS, is being developed as related to naturally occurring vitamins and nutrients. The NOS will also help to support a platform for a program of related research and development to establish a "Naturally Occurring Daily Intake" that may be established as a quantitative consumer guide and standard for naturally occurring vitamins and nutrients as an alternative reference to the current RDI and DV standards that refer primarily to synthetic vitamins and nutrients.

Introduction

As director/practitioner at the Hippocrates Health Institute, a residential therapeutic center where patients generally reside for 21 days, I pioneered clinical research directly relating to the absorbability of supplemental nutrients. For the past 20 years, we have observed 18,000 patients' blood microscopically. From this emerged 11,750 individuals who were consuming one or many varieties of isolated chemical nutritional supplements.

We found it to be almost unanimous that these cases showed little to no absorption of any of these purported nutrients. This determination was easily made with acute observation of crystalline particulate in the blood. Dr. Treadway and I consider this to be of paramount concern and have moved forward with further research and concrete plans to establish whole-food nutrient standards that will lay the groundwork in differentiating chemical versus whole and thorough effectiveness versus the often irrelevant, stimulating, or depressing effects laboratory derived nutrients provoke.

Background and Discussion

Production of synthetic vitamins began in earnest in the late 1930s and 1940s and today the majority of vitamin dietary supplements and vitamin-fortified foods commercially available are derived from synthetics. These synthetic vitamins are manmade in chemical laboratories and are not from nature, although the product labeling of these substances is often associated with the word *natural*. For example, some vitamin products that use synthetic vitamins may have a label that indicates "natural." Part of this use of the word *natural* may be due to the fact that a legal "natural" label designation under some provisions and conditions may be permitted when there is at least a 10 percent natural base of food or botanicals in the product and therefore, this use may represent an abuse of the word.

The older RDAs (Recommended Dietary Allowances) and current DVs (Daily Values), as related to synthetic vitamins and supported by our government, tend to perpetuate the use of synthetic vitamins and the notion that synthetic vitamins are somehow "natural" based upon the assumption that synthetic nutrient chemical structures are similar to those found in nature. Isolated chemical compounds that resemble parts of complete, complex vitamin factors are *not* the same as real, complex vitamins in their full matrix as found in nature. In this way, the NOS will challenge the definition of what a "vitamin" really is.

The history of vitamins and nutrients points to the origin of vitamin use for vitamin deficiency diseases before there was a modern understanding of what a vitamin is. Hundreds of years ago, as a practical matter, the British Navy discovered that the ingestion of limes or other citrus fruit by their naval personnel was useful to prevent scurvy, which we now know as a vitamin C deficiency disease. Before the British Navy implemented the regular use of citrus fruit to prevent scurvy there was a large-percentage loss of British naval personnel each year to the dreaded disease. Similar situations related to deficiency diseases, such as pellagra or beriberi, which we now know as vitamin B deficiency conditions, were prevented by the use of rice polish and were established historical treatments of vitamin deficiency diseases. Later, when chemical analysis of foods and their compounds became available, it was discovered that certain foods contained "vitamins," or complex groups of natural compounds that were responsible for the biological action that prevented specific vitamin deficiency diseases. This brings us to the question of what a vitamin really is. Can a vitamin be defined as only one or two active compounds found in a food and then be chemically copied and medically administered with an expectation that the supposed copied vitamin is the whole vitamin? Is it just an isolated fraction?

An assumption of the NOS is that all synthetic vitamins are not natural and are only parts (fractions) of a whole vitamin. This means that a part cannot be the whole, and a fraction of a vitamin is not a real, whole vitamin, but only part of the whole vitamin matrix. For example, many assume that ascorbic acid, a part of the whole vitamin known as vitamin C, is actually vitamin C, and so they call ascorbic acid "vitamin C." Ascorbic acid is an important *component* of vitamin C, but there are other components, and therefore ascorbic acid is not vitamin C. Ascorbic acid is only a part of a complete matrix known as vitamin C. The phrase "vitamin C" came about after Albert Szent-Györgyi, the Nobel Prize winner, isolated a substance from the adrenal glands. He called it hexuronic acid. At around the same time, W.A. Waugh and Charles King isolated a vitamin from lemon and showed that it was nearly identical to hexuronic acid. In 1932, this vitamin, known as vitamin C, became the first (fraction of a vitamin) to be synthesized in a laboratory. Real, whole vitamin C is not only ascorbic acid, but includes a matrix of compounds, some known, such as bioflavonoids and tannins, and some that are still unknown.

Synthetic vitamins and nutrients have been shown to exhibit toxic effects when ingested. These toxic reactions are similar to some adverse drug reactions, or "side effects," often associated with drugs that are also synthetic chemical compounds. The adverse effects of large doses of synthetic vitamin E, synthetic carotene, synthetic vitamin D, synthetic vitamin C, and many other synthetic nutrients is well known. The fact that there is a distinction between synthetic vitamins and nutrients and "natural" or naturally occurring vitamins and nutrients is accepted and recognized by various institutions and organizations, and also by certain large commercial pharmaceutical corporations who manufacture synthetic vitamins and nutrients and who rightfully support the restriction of these substances in the same manner as drugs are restricted.

Although there is currently no official, U.S. government–regulated definition for the term *natural* pertaining to the natural products industry, the Food and Drug Administration (FDA) refers to natural ingredients as "ingredients extracted directly from plants or animal products as opposed to being produced synthetically."

We support the FDA statement, especially as related to the distinction between natural (naturally occurring) and synthetic vitamins and nutrients. We also agree with a statement from the Codex Alimentarius court proceedings as conducted in Europe related to the definition of natural vitamins as opposed to synthetic vitamins and nutrients as reported by the Alliance for Natural Health on July 12, 2005, and partially represented and quoted as follows:

> The ban on non-positive list of vitamins and minerals does not apply at all to vitamins and minerals normally found in or consumed as part of the diet which therefore are not banned as of 1 August 2005. Where the FSD does apply (which is to vitamins and minerals derived from 'chemical substances' i.e. not naturally derived). Court has stated that the Directive is to be interpreted as applying only to 'food supplements containing vitamins and/or minerals derived from a manufacturing process using "chemical substances,"' not other food supplements (paragraph 63 of the judgment).

It is evident that there is recognition by FDA and the legal associates of Codex Alimentarius among other highly recognized authorities, institutions, and corporations globally who recognize that there is a definite distinction between natural (naturally occurring) vitamins and nutrients and synthetic vitamins and nutrients. The knowledge of the distinction between natural and synthetic vitamins and nutrients, although recognized by certain leading persons and organizations in the food industry, seems to be missing from the general public domain, and therefore this knowledge needs to be brought forward in a broad public manner and disseminated in an organized program of public awareness and education. The establishment of the NOS will help to support such a consumer education program.

The NOS, as proposed, is a standard that may be used to certify food and food supplement potencies for vitamins and other nutrients. The potencies of fortified food, vitamin, and nutrient products once certified as "NOS" would indicate to the end user or consumer that the products or raw materials in question contain labeled potencies of nutrients that are derived only from naturally occurring, food-derived sources. This certification process might be similar in structure to the current certification protocols associated with "organic" foods. However, the difference for the NOS certification, as opposed to other certification programs, such as the "organic food" certification program, is that the NOS certification of food and food supplement products will be focused upon the distinction between natural vitamins and nutrients and synthetic vitamins and nutrients.

Certification will depend upon the exclusive use of only naturally occurring nutrients and their potencies as derived strictly from naturally occurring, food-derived sources being used in the raw materials or finished food products and labeled accordingly. As an example of how the NOS would work as a certification tool for vitamin supplements we should first observe the current situation. Most commercially available vitamin supplement lines today use some synthesized forms of vitamins or nutrient materials added directly or indirectly (spiked in a medium such as yeast or other materials). NOS-certified supplements would, presumably, contain no synthetic nutrients of any kind, added directly or indirectly. An NOS-certified vitamin and nutrient product would tend to have listed potencies that would be generally quantitatively lower-potency, based upon current standards such as RDIs and DVs, than synthetic-containing products due to the nature of popular high-potency vitamin supplements that are dependent upon synthetic quantities. These synthetic-potency products are often manipulated to reflect higher concentrations of nutrient potencies (synthetic potencies) than are found naturally occurring in foods or food and botanical concentrates.

The difference between products that contain vitamin and nutrient potencies derived from synthetics and those potencies that are naturally occurring can be distinguished on a product label through the process of NOS certification and logo attachment upon the labeled product, allowing the end user or consumer to choose between NOS (naturally occurring nutrient–containing) and non-NOS (synthetic nutrient–containing) products.

Any NOS certified supplement product would be expected to mention the phrase *naturally occurring* or the equivalent on the label when referring to the labeled potency claim(s), and should reference the food or botanical source of the claimed naturally occurring source. If either of these pieces of information is missing from the vitamin, nutrient, or mineral food supplement or fortified food label related to any particular nutrient, then a consumer could be fairly confident that the product potencies of the vitamins, for example the B vitamins, are synthetic and not naturally occurring or derived only from naturally occurring food sources. There may be many more details and exceptions to consider, but the NOS certification approach will provide a general guide to help the health professional or consumer distinguish between natural and synthetic vitamin and nutrient products and materials.

Because of the mass marketing of synthetic vitamins as "natural," or the equivalent of real, natural vitamins throughout the last 70 years, the general public has become confused about real, natural vitamins as opposed to those that are synthetic. The significant difference between real, natural vitamins and nutrients, as made by nature, and manmade synthetic vitamins and nutrients can be the difference between healthy nutrition and disease-causing toxicity.

Today the vast majority of vitamins ingested through vitamin supplementation and fortified foods are synthetic compounds made in a laboratory and divorced from nature. Synthetic vitamins are similar to drugs because they are synthesized chemical compounds. Many synthetic vitamin compounds have proven to have toxic side effects. For example, it has been found that synthetic vitamin A can cause birth defects, and studies on synthesized beta-carotene (provitamin A) have shown that this synthetic "vitamin" may contribute to heart attacks and cancers. Similar studies on the side effects of synthetic vitamin E illustrate the point that synthetic vitamins have a net negative effect on health. Although synthetic vitamins may be used as drugs for successful emergency treatment, many who support natural vitamin and nutrient supplementation oppose synthetic vitamin and nutrient use for long-term daily intake.

Supporters of truly natural vitamins and nutrients historically have been opposed to the development of the synthetic vitamin and nutrient paradigm, citing the dangers of allowing synthetic vitamins and nutrients to enter our mainstream processed foods and supplementation market. One of the pioneers and noteworthy proponents of naturally occurring vitamins and nutrients was Dr. Royal Lee, who used his personal time and resources to relate the problems associated with synthetic vitamins to educate the public on the dangers of synthetic vitamins. He also presented his research and made his case for the avoidance of synthetic nutrients to the commercial food processing industry and to associated U.S. government agencies.

Because synthetic vitamins may be viewed as toxic chemical compounds similar to drugs, the establishment of the NOS and NOS certification of products becomes urgent and vital for the identification of natural products. It is also critical for the self-regulation and protection of our food supplement industry and the consumers who support it. This is also a timely consideration due to the encroachment of draconian legislation efforts aimed at the control of all synthetic nutrients.

Summary

Today there are two main categories of vitamin supplements generally available commercially. They are as follows:

1. Supplements containing chemical vitamins (such as USP manmade vitamins or nutrients) added to a natural base. This category is related to the *direct* addition of synthetic vitamins and nutrients to a product and represents a majority of the supplements and fortified foods available today.

2. "Food Grown" or "Food Based" supplements. In this category, product potencies are often derived by adding

(spiking) chemical, synthetic vitamins and nutrients into a base such as yeast, algae, other bacteriums, or a mixture of various materials, and then using that artificially potentized (spiked) material base or a portion of that base for all or part of the labeled potency of the product.

These labeled products may have a generally misleading claim, referring to the spiked base as the "food" source. (This category represents the *indirect* addition of synthetic vitamins and nutrients.) The indirect addition of synthetic nutrients, in this case, is apparently for label claims of "Food Source," which can be legally made if the base that the synthetics are added to (spiked into or "grown" within, such as yeast or other materials) is referred to as natural "food." The establishment of the NOS will help to create a new category of NOS vitamin and nutrient food supplements that represent a food-inherent, naturally occurring vitamin and/or nutrient food supplement, bulk food material, or fortified food, with labeled potencies derived only from food and botanical extract sources with related, labeled, and assayed potency values.

All NOS supplement potencies, as labeled, will be derived directly from food and botanical concentrates with a minimum quantitative standard. The NOS certification cannot be issued if synthetic vitamins, inorganic minerals, or synthetic nutrients of any kind have been added to the NOS supplement applicant product either directly or indirectly.

The NOS may be developed and used by the food industry as a consumer standard for all food supplements or fortified foods. The NOS symbol printed on dietary supplements or food product labels will alert the consumer that the product has only naturally occurring nutrient values and verified potencies. This will help the consumer to make a more informed choice.

Conclusion

In order to remove public confusion and to clarify what real vitamins and nutrients are as opposed to synthetic vitamins and nutrients, we propose using the NOS standard for the food and food supplement industry and for every producer of a food or a food supplement product, as well as for every nutritional or botanical product. Our proposal is aimed at bringing a full disclosure to the consumer. In this regard, we propose that any time a vitamin content or potency is claimed in a food or food supplement product, the label should clearly state if the vitamin or nutrient is "naturally occurring" or not. The term *naturally occurring vitamin* (or *nutrient*) such as *naturally occurring vitamin A*, should not be used on the product label if, in fact, the vitamin or nutrient is not naturally occurring within the product ingredients as claimed on the label. In this manner, it then can be understood by the consumer that if the product ingredient(s) do not contain vitamins or nutrients that are "naturally occurring," then it may be assumed that these ingredients have been added or "fortified" into the product, and that these fortified synthetic chemical versions of vitamins and nutrients may be understood as distinctly non-natural as opposed to any naturally occurring vitamins and nutrients.

APPENDIX C

RESOURCES FOR NATURAL PRODUCTS

The following is a list of links and sources for real, naturally occurring vitamins, NOS food supplements, and NOS ingredients and information.

Alliance for Natural Health (NOS Approaches)
Unit 5, Forge End
St. Albans, Hertfordshire
AL2 3EQ United Kingdom
www.alliance-natural-health.org
44 (0) 1252 371 275
info@alliance-natural-health.org

Amsarusa (NOS Standards & Products)
10336 Loch Lomond Rd. #233
Loch Lomond, CA 95461
www.amsarusa.com

Big Tree Health Products (NOS Products)
P.O. Box 438 Sedgefield
6573 South Africa
www.bigtreehealth.com

Metaorganics
(Naturally Occurring Medicinal Botanical Supplements)
www.metaorganics.net
(800) 584–3533

Naturally Occurring Standards Group (NOSG)
www.nosg.org
(775) 540–0457

Botani Organics Naturally Occurring Vitamin Supplements
www.alohabay.com
(800) 994–3267

Hippocrates Health Institute (NOS Products)
1443 Palmdale Ct.
West Palm Beach, FL 33411
www.hippocratesinst.com
(561) 471–8876

The Weston A. Price Foundation (NOS Approaches)
PMB 106-380, 4200 Wisconsin Ave., NW
Washington, DC 20016
www.westonaprice.org
(202) 333–HEAL
westonaprice@msn.com

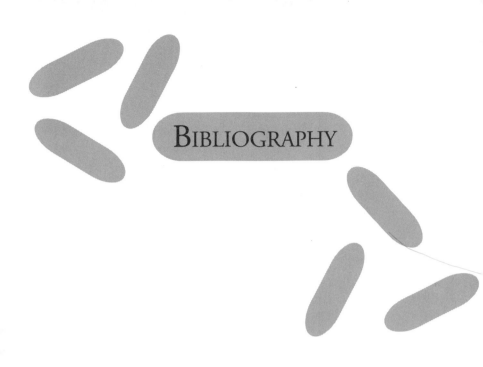

BIBLIOGRAPHY

Acuff, R.V. "Vitamin E: bioavailability and function of natural and synthetic forms." *American Journal of Natural Medicine* 5:10–13, 59 (1998).

"Alliance for Natural Health Critiques JAMA Study." March 5, 2007. *www.alliance-natural-health.org* (accessed 8/12/09).

"Alpha Tocopherol Beta Carotene Cancer Prevention Study Group, The." National Cancer Institute. *http://dceg.cancer.gov/atbcstudy/study_details.html* (accessed 8/12/09).

Bernard-Gallon, D.J. et al. "Differential effects of *n*-3 and *n*-6 polyunsaturated fatty acids on *BRCA1* and *BRCA2* gene expression in breast cell lines." *British Journal of Nutrition* 87(4):281–9 (April 1, 2002).

Bjelakovic, G., et al. "Mortality in Randomized Trials of Antioxidant Supplements for Primary and Secondary Prevention: Systematic Review and Meta-Analysis." *JAMA* 297:842–57 (February 28, 2007).

Blumberg, Jeffrey. "Unraveling the Conflicting Studies on Vitamin E and Heart Disease." Linus Pauling Institute, Oregon State University. May 2002. *http:// lpi.oregonstate.edu/ss02/blumberg.html* (accessed 8/12/09).

Booth, S.L., J.A. Pennington, and J.A. Sadowski. "Food sources and dietary intakes of Vitamin K-1 (phylloquinone) in the American diet: Data from the FDA Total Diet Study." *Journal of the American Dietetic Association* 96(2):149–54 (February 1996).

Borenstein, B. "Vitamin Fortification Technology" in *Technology of Fortification of Foods.* Washington, D.C.: National Academy of Sciences, 1975.

Brehm, W. "Potential dangers of viosterol during pregnancy with observations of calcification of placentae." *Ohio State Medical Journal* 33(9):989–993 (September 1937), as reviewed by *Modern Medicine,* October 1937, p. 62.

Brophy, Beth, and David Schardt. "Functional Foods." Center for Science in the Public Interest. April 1999. *http:// cspinet.org/nah/4_99/functional_foods.htm* (accessed 8/12/09).

Burton, G.W. "Human plasma and tissue a-tochopherol concentrations in response to supplementation with deuterated natural and synthetic vitamin E." *American Journal of Clinical Nutrition* 67:669–84 (1998).

Campbell, Joseph D. "Minerals and Disease." *The Journal of Orthomolecular Medicine* 10, No. 3 & 4 (1995).

Campbell, T. Colin. "RDAs: Time to Peel Back the Labels." September 2005. *www.nutritionadvocate.com/story/ rdas.htm* (accessed 8/12/09).

"CDC: Few Americans meet fruit, veggie guidelines." Associated Press. March 15, 2007.

Challem, J.J. "Beta-carotene and Other Carotenoids: Promises, Failures and a New Vision." *The Journal of Orthomolecular Medicine* 12:11–19 (1st Quarter 1997).

Challem, Jack. "The Past, Present and Future of Vitamins." *The Nutrition Reporter*, 1997.

Clement, Brian R. *Living Foods for Optimum Health*. New York: Three Rivers Press, 1998.

Clement, Brian R., PhD, NMD, LNC. *Hippocrates Life Force: Superior Health & Longevity*. Summertown, Tenn.: Healthy Living Publication, 2007.

Crawford, Alan Pell. "What does 'natural' mean?" *Vegetarian Times*, September 2004.

"CRN Urges Government to Provide Consumers With More Realistic Nutrition Advice." September 21, 2004. Council for Responsible Nutrition, *www.crnusa.org* (accessed 8/12/09).

DeCava, Judith. *The Real Truth About Vitamins and Antioxidants*. Columbus, Ga.: Brentwood Academy Press, 1996.

Dietary Guidelines for Americans, 2005. *www.healthierus.gov/ dietaryguidelines* (accessed 8/12/09).

Docherty, John, et al. "A Double-Blind, Placebo-Controlled Exploratory Trial of Chromium Picolinate in Atypical Depression." *The Journal of Psychiatric Practice* 11, Issue 5 (September 2005).

Dr. Rona's Healthwise Digest. March 18, 2007. *http:// drzoltanrona.typepad.com* (accessed 8/12/09).

Earth Summit 1992. UN Conference on Environment and Development. *www.un.org/geninfo/bp/enviro.html* (accessed 8/12/09).

"The Effect of Vitamin E and Beta Carotene on the Incidence of Lung Cancer and Other Cancer in Male Smokers." Beta Carotene Cancer Prevention Study Group. *New England Journal of Medicine* 330 (15):1029–35 (April 14, 1994).

Fairfield, K.M., and R.H. Fletcher. "Vitamins for Chronic Disease Prevention in Adults." *Journal of the American Medical Association* 287:3116–26 (2002).

Feher, Miklos, and Jonathan M. Schmidt. "Differences Between Drugs, Natural Products, and Molecules From Combinatorial Chemistry." *Journal of Chemical Information and Computer Science* 43(1): 218–27 (2003).

Fickova, M., P. Hubert, G. Cremel, and C. Leray. "Dietary *n*-3 and *n*-6 polyunsaturated fatty acids rapidly modify fatty acid composition and insulin effects in rat adipocytes." *Journal of Nutrition* 128(3):512–19 (March 1, 1998).

Fitzgerald, Randall. *The Hundred Year Lie: How Food and Medicine Are Destroying Your Health.* New York: Penguin/Dutton, 2006.

Frost, Mary. *Going Back to the Basics of Human Health.* San Diego, Calif.: International Foundation for Nutrition and Health, 1997.

Griffith, H. Winter, MD. *Minerals, Supplements & Vitamins: The Essential Guide.* Cambridge, Mass.: Da Capo Press, 2000.

Groff, J.L., S.S. Gropper, and S.M. Hunt. *Advanced Nutrition and Human Metabolism.* New York: West Publishing Company, 1995.

Hays, G.L., et al. "Salivary pH while dissolving vitamin C-containing tablets." *American Journal of Dentistry* 5(5): 269–71 (October 1992).

Heber, Dr. David, "Testimony Before the House Government Reform Committee." July 25, 2002. *www.cancercurecoalition.org/articles/ nutritionandcancer.html* (accessed 8/12/09).

Heller, A. and T. Koch. "Immunonutrition with omega-3-fatty acids: Are new anti-inflammatory strategies in sight?" *Zentralblatt fur Chirurgie* 125(2):123–36 (2000).

Hellerman, Caleb. "No scientific evidence diet supplements work." *www.cnn.com/2007/HEALTH/04/06/ chasing.supplements/index.html?iref=newssearch.* Atlanta, Ga., April 16, 2007 (accessed 8/12/09).

Hilton, J.W., and S.J. Slinger. "Nutrition and feeding of rainbow trout." *Canadian Special Publication of Fisheries and Aquatic Sciences* 55:15 (1981).

Hoffer, Abram. "Playing with Statistics or Lies, Damn Lies and Statistics." *The Journal of Orthomolecular Medicine* 13:67–71 (2nd Quarter 1998).

Howell, E. *Enzyme Nutrition.* Wayne, N.J.: Avery Publishing, 1985.

Hurley, Dan. *Natural Causes: Death, Lies, and Politics in America's Vitamin and Herbal Supplement Industry.* New York: Broadway Books, 2006.

Jacobson, Michael F., and David Schardt. "Diet, ADHD & Behavior." The Center for Science in the Public Interest, September 1999. *www.cspinet.org* (accessed 8/12/09).

Jenkins D.J.A., T.M.S. Wolever, and A.L. Jenkins. "Diet Factors Affecting Nutrient Absorption and Metabolism," in *Modern Nutrition in Health and Disease,* 8th ed. Lea and Phil Febiger, 1994 (583–602).

Jennings, Isobel. *Vitamins in Endocrine Metabolism.* London: Heinemann Medical, 1970.

Lawson, Stephen. "Recent Research on Vitamins C and E." Oregon State University, Linus Pauling Institute, Spring/Summer 2005 Research Report.

Lee, Dr. Royal, "What Is a Vitamin?" *Applied Trophology* (August 1956).

Lieberman, Shari, PhD. *The Real Vitamin & Mineral Book.* New York: Penguin Group, 2003.

"A little risky business." *The Economist.* Nov. 22, 2007. *www.economist.com/science/ displaystory.cfm?story_id=E1_TDTSTNTN* (accessed 8/24/09).

Madley, Rebecca H. *Nutraceuticals World* 7:58 (July 4, 2001).

Mason-Scarborough, Dr. Laura. "Vitamins—Synthetic vs. Natural." July 18, 2004. Holistic Pediatric Association. *www.hpakids.org/holistic-health* (accessed 8/12/09).

"Modern Miracle Men" U.S. Senate Document #264, June 1936.

Moss, R.W. *Free Radical—Albert Szent-Györgyi and the Battle Over Vitamin C*. New York: Paragon House, 1988.

"Nanoparticles in Sun Creams Can Stress Brain Cells." *www.nature.com*. Published online June 16, 2006; doi:10.1038/news060612-14.

"Natural or Whole Food Supplements vs. Isolated Chemical Compounds." Organic Consumers Association, March 2007. *www.organicconsumers.org/nutricon/qa.cfm* (accessed 8/12/09).

"Natural Vitamin E vs. Synthetic." *Townsend Letter for Doctors & Patients*, July 1999.

Nestle, Marion. *Food Politics*. Berkeley, Calif.: University of California Press, 2003.

"Nutri-Con: The Truth About Vitamins and Supplements." Organic Consumer's Association, 2007. *www.organicconsumers.org* (accessed 8/12/09).

O'Halloran, Thomas, et al. "Metal Ion Chaperone Function of the Soluble Cu(I) Receptor Atx1." *Science* 278, No. 5339, 853–56 (October 1997).

O'Shea, Tim. "Whole Food Vitamins: Ascorbic Acid Is Not Vitamin C." *www.whale.to/a/shea1.html* (accessed 8/12/09).

Pollan, Michael. "Unhappy Meals." *The New York Times*, January 28, 2007.

Price, Weston. *Nutrition and Physical Degeneration*. New Canaan, Conn.: Keats Pub., 1997.

Quinlivan, Eoin, and Jesse F. Gregory III. "Effect of food fortification on folic acid intake in the United States." *American Journal of Clinical Nutrition* 77, No. 1, 221–5 (January 2003).

Randolph, Theron, MD. *Human Ecology and Susceptibility to the Chemical Environment (7th ed.)*. Springfield, Ill.: Charles C. Thomas Publisher, 1980.

Recommended Dietary Allowances, 10th Edition. Washington, D.C.: National Academy Press Food and Nutrition Board, 2000.

Schroeder, H.A. *The Trace Elements and Man.* New Greenwich, Conn.: Devin-Adair, 1973.

Severus, W.E., A.B. Littman, and A.L. Stoll. "Omega-3 fatty acids, homocysteine, and the increased risk of cardiovascular mortality in major depressive disorder." *Harvard Review of Psychiatry* 9(6):280–93 (Nov.–Dec. 2001).

Sexton, Timothy. "Your Guide to Vitamin Supplements." *www.associatedcontent.com/subject/article/ your+guide+to+vitamin+supplements,* August 7, 2005 (accessed 8/12/09).

Shimek, Ronald, PhD. "The Toxicity of Some Freshly Mixed Artificial Sea Water." *Reefkeeping Online Magazine* (1999). *www.reefkeeping.com* (accessed 8/12/09).

Smythies, John. "Recent Advances in Oxidative Stress and Antioxidants in Medicine." *Journal of Orthomolecular Medicine* 13(1):11–18 (1998).

Sourer (1995); Whitney, et al. (1996); Sizer, et al. (1997). "Calcium Functions." National Research Council.

"Statement of Assistant Attorney General Joel I. Klein." May 20, 1999. U.S. Department of Justice. *www.usdoj.gov/ atr/public/press_releases/1999/2451.pdf* (accessed 8/12/09).

Stoll, B.A. "N-3 fatty acids and lipid peroxidation in breast cancer inhibition." *British Journal of Nutrition* 87(3):193–8 (March 2002).

"Study Citing Antioxidant Vitamin Risks Based on Flawed Methodology." Linus Pauling Institute, February 27, 2007. *www.oregonstate.edu/dept/ncs/newsarch/2007/ Feb07/vitaminstudy.html* (accessed 8/12/09).

Supplee, G., S. Ansbacher, R. Bender, and G. Flanigan. "The Influence of Milk Constituents on the Effectiveness of Vitamin D." *Journal of Biological Chemistry* 114:95–107 (May 1936).

Traber, M.G., et al. "Synthetic as compared with natural vitamin E is preferentially excreted as á-CEHC in human urine: Studies using deuterated á-tocopheryl acetates." *FEBS Letters* 437(1):145–148 (October 16, 1998).

"The Truth About Vitamins" Australian Broadcasting Corporation. March 24, 2005. *www.abc.net.au* (accessed 8/12/09).

U.S. Dietary Guidelines. *www.health.gov/DietaryGuidelines* (accessed 8/12/09).

U.S. FDA. "Definition of Natural." Consumer Information & Publication No. 95–5012. November 1991; revised May 1995. *www.usda.gov* (accessed 8/12/09).

Vinson, J.A., P. Bose. "Bioavailability of Synthetic Ascorbic Acid and a Citrus Extract." *Annals of the New York Academy of Sciences, 3rd Conference on Vitamin C* 498, 525–6 (1987).

Vinson, J.A. "Comparative Bioavailability of Synthetic and Natural Vitamin C in Guinea Pigs." *Nutrition Reports International* 27(4): 875–80 (1983).

"Vitamin E Might Make Heart Disease Worse." Associated Press, November 10, 2004.

Waisman, Harry A., and C.A. Elvehjem. "Multiple Deficiencies in the Modified Goldberger Diet as Demonstrated With Chicks." Department of Chemistry, College of Agriculture, University of Wisconsin, Madison. *http://jn.nutrition.org/cgi/reprint/20/6/519.pdf* (accessed 08/27/09).

Wallace, R.A. *Biology: The World of Life*, 6th ed. New York: HarperCollins, 1992.

Watkins, B.A., Y. Li, and M.F. Seifert. "Nutraceutical Fatty Acids as Biochemical and Molecular Modulators of Skeletal Biology." *Journal of the American College of Nutrition* 20(90005):410S–416S (October 1, 2001).

Watkins, B.A., Y. Li, H.E. Lippman, and M.F. Seifert. "Omega-3 Polyunsaturated Fatty Acids and Skeletal Health." *Experimental Biology and Medicine* (Maywood) 226(6):485–97 (June 2001).

Winter, Ruth. *Consumer's Dictionary of Food Additives.* New York: Three Rivers Press, 2004.

Wu, M., et al. "Omega-3 polyunsaturated fatty acids attenuate breast cancer growth through activation of a neutral sphingomyelinase-mediated pathway." *International Journal of Cancer* 117(3):340–48 (September 21, 2005).

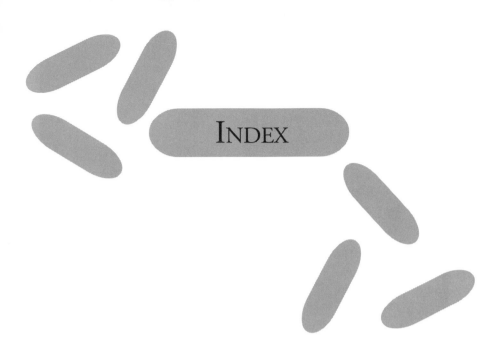

INDEX

ABOUT THE AUTHOR

DR. BRIAN CLEMENT, PhD, NMD, LN, pioneered the international progressive health movement. Now in his fourth decade of research, directorship, lecturing, and investigating, he is renowned in the field of authentic medicine. Utilizing a wide cross-section of lifestyle methods and non-invasive technologies including both the consumption of whole-food supplements and the intravenous process, he has become the leading authority on supplementation and the orthomolecular effect it has on prevention and recovery. Dr. Clement and his team are on a constant quest to expand the parameters in the elimination of disease and premature aging. His Florida center has pioneered a program and established training in active aging and longevity. With hundreds of thousands of people participating in this program in the last half century, volumes of data have been accrued, giving Clement a privileged insight into the lifestyle required to maintain youth, vitality, and stamina. Among all of Dr. Clement's many contributions, he is proudest of *Supplements Exposed*, because he knows it will open the eyes of millions and protect them from the ill effects that most of these pills and potions create.